FOOT
AND
ANKLE PAIN

RENE CAILLIET, M.D.

Chief of Department of Physical Medicine
Southern California Permanente Medical Group
Los Angeles

Clinical Professor
University of Southern California School of Medicine
Department of Physical Medicine and Rehabilitation

Department Head, Physical Medicine
Kaiser Foundation Hospitals, Southern California

F. A. DAVIS COMPANY *Philadelphia*

Also by Rene Cailliet:

LOW BACK PAIN SYNDROME

SHOULDER PAIN

NECK AND ARM PAIN

HAND: PAIN AND IMPAIRMENT

Library of Congress Catalog Card Number 67-29296
ISBN-0-8036-1600-7

Preface

Man's foot is subjected to daily stresses and strains. It is cramped into ill-fitting shoes, made to walk on hard surfaces, and allowed to become debilitated by constant trauma and misuse. The study of the bones and muscles of the foot during medical training is too often presented in an uninteresting and confusing manner with no correlation to function. Care of the ailing foot is then relegated to the unscientifically trained shoe salesman or boot maker.

The foot presents a segment of the human anatomy that is accessible to examination, palpation, and complete mechanical evaluation. No portion of the foot escapes the discerning eye if the functional anatomy is clearly understood.

The history given by the patient describes misuse of the foot, and the examination verifies the mechanism causing the pain. As in previous volumes, on *Low Back Pain, Neck and Arm Pain,* and *Shoulder Pain,* the first portion of this book is devoted to normal functional anatomy. Subsequent chapters discuss various painful conditions and how each is related to the abnormal mechanism causing the pain and disability. Logical treatment which attempts to correct or alter the abnormality discovered from the history and physical examination is described.

My sincere thanks is expressed to my associate Dr. Lionel Jacobs who spent many hours documenting many of the statements and literally rewrote many sections of the book. Again, my sincere appreciation is expressed to Dr. Sidney Licht and the physicians of the Gaylord Seminar, Drs. Frederick Dugdale, Thomas F. Hines, Ian MacLean, Krystyna Piertorwska, Herman L. Kamenetz, and Sung Liao, who read the manuscript and made many valuable suggestions. Mere words cannot express my gratitude to my wife for her patience and assistance in compiling the final writing.

RENE CAILLIET, M.D.

Table of Contents

iv

Illustrations

CHAPTER 1

Structural Anatomy

The foot is a complex unit composed of twenty-six bones that can bear the full-body weight on standing and is able to transport the human body over all kinds of terrain. The twenty-six bones consist of fourteen phalanges, five metatarsals, and seven tarsal bones. The foot can be divided into three functional segments (Fig. 1). The posterior segment lies directly under the tibia and supports it. This segment contains (1) the talus at the apex of the foot which is a part of the ankle joint, and (2) the calcaneus which is the hind portion of the foot and in contact with the ground. The middle segment contains five tarsal bones which form an irregular rhomboid with medial base and lateral apex. The three cuneiforms and the anterior part of the cuboid form a row with the navicular bone and the posterior portion of the cuboid behind. The anterior segment of the foot contains five metatarsal and fourteen phalangeal bones. The big toe has two phalanges, whereas the outer toes contain three each.

OSSEOUS COMPONENTS

The foot can best be understood structurally and functionally if each bone is related in position and movement to the others. The *talus* is the mechanical keystone at the apex of the foot. It has a body, a neck, and a head. The superior surface and both sides of the body support and articulate with the tibia and fibula. The convex, saddle-shaped, superior surface of the talus glides under the tibia during ankle motion (Fig. 2).

The two sides and the superior surface of the talus are covered with articular cartilage and are "gripped" between the malleoli and tibia which form the ankle mortice. The tibial malleolus extends about one third of the way down the medial surface of the body of the talus, whereas the fibular malleolus covers its entire lateral surface. The superior portion of the body supports the tibia. Within this mortice, the talus functions as a hinge joint.

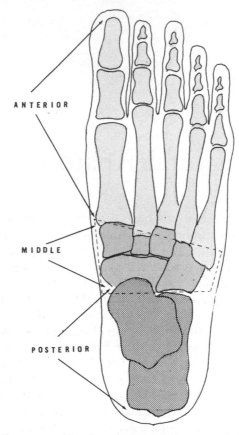

FIGURE 1.   The three functional segments of the foot.

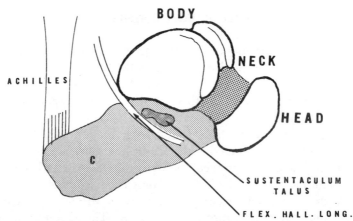

FIGURE 2.   Talus. The talus is at the apex of the posterior segment of the foot. It is divisible into a body, neck, and head. The body has two articular surfaces that fit into the ankle mortice. The head articulates with the middle segment, and the entire talus fits upon and articulates with the calcaneus.

When viewed from above, the ankle mortice is laterally angled since the medial malleolus is anterior to the lateral malleolus in the transverse plane (Fig. 3). The body of the talus is wedge shaped with the wider portion anterior (Fig. 4). As the ankle dorsiflexes, this wider portion comes up between the two malleoli and wedges between them. Plantar flexion of the foot presents the posterior narrower portion of the talus between the malleoli and in this position permits some lateral motion of the talus within the mortice. This mobility creates instability of the joint and places an added burden on its supporting ligaments.

LIGAMENTS

Ligaments provide further stability to the ankle joint. The integrity of the ankle mortice is maintained by the interosseous ligament and membrane and the anterior and posterior tibiofibular ligaments. The interosseous ligament attaches to the inner aspect of the tibia and proceeds laterally and downward to the inner aspect of the fibula. The fibula rises slightly during ankle dorsiflexion (Fig. 5) and causes the fibers to become more nearly horizontal thus widening the mortice as the wider portion of the talus enters it. With full dorsiflexion the mortice is fully expanded, and further dorsiflexion is checked. Plantar flexion presents the narrower portion of the talus within the mortice, and the fibula rides down returning the interosseous ligament to its oblique course. The mortice here is narrower. The interosseous ligament and membrane is reinforced by the posterior and anterior tibiofibular ligaments that run parallel to the interosseous ligament. These ligaments may be torn in severe ankle sprains and fractures.

The ankle joint receives its strongest support from the collateral ligaments. The lateral collateral ligament supports the lateral aspect of the ankle and is composed of three bands: (a) the anterior talofibular ligament which originates on the neck of the talus and attaches to the tip of the fibula, (b) the calcaneofibular ligament which runs from the calcaneus to the tip of the fibula, and (c) the posterior talofibular ligament which runs from the body of the talus to the tip of the fibula (Fig. 6).

The anterior talofibular and the calcaneofibular ligaments are the ones most frequently injured when the ankle is sprained. This is usually an inversion injury while the ankle is in its most unstable position, that of plantar flexion.

The medial aspect of the ankle joint is strongly supported by the deltoid ligament which courses from the medial malleolus to the navicular, the sustentaculum talus, and the posterior aspect of the talus. The deltoid ligament is composed of four bands: (1) the tibionavicular, (2) the anterior talotibial, (3) the calcaneotibial, and (4) the posterior talotibial. The deltoid ligament is so strong that severe eversion stress upon the ankle

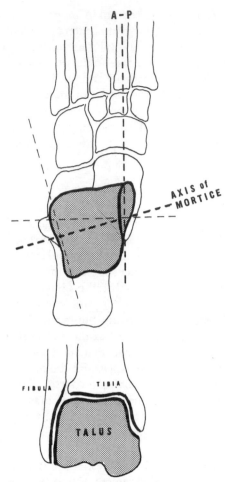

FIGURE 3. Superior view of the talus. Viewed from above the talus is wedge shaped being wider anteriorly. It fits between the tibial and fibular malleoli that form the ankle mortice.

will usually cause avulsion of the malleolus rather than a tear of this ligament.

Dorsiflexion and plantar flexion of the ankle occur about an axis which passes transversely through the body of the talus (Fig. 3 and 4). The lateral end of the ankle axis passes through the tip of the fibula and is centrally located between the attachments of the lateral collateral ligaments (Fig. 7) allowing them to remain taut during all movements. At its medial end the transverse axis is placed eccentrically to the point of attachment of the medial ligaments. In this situation the posterior medial ligaments become taut on dorsiflexion and the anterior medial ligaments

4

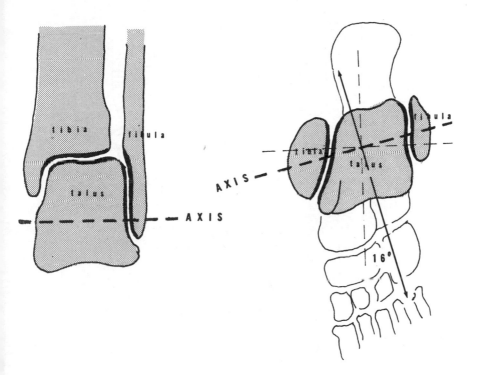

FIGURE 4. Ankle mortice and talus relationship. The axis of rotation within the mortice as the ankle plantar and dorsiflexes is shown on the left. It passes through the fibula but below the tip of the tibia. Viewed from above the tibia is anterior to the fibula forming an external "toe out" of 16 degrees.

become tight on plantar flexion. This arrangement of alternating tightness and slackness restricts the range of plantar and dorsal motion of the ankle.

The talocalcaneal joint (the subtalar joint) contains several joints in different planes which permit simultaneous movements in different directions. The talocalcaneal joint is divided into two synovial lined chambers by an oblique canal formed by a groove in the talus and a corresponding groove in the calcaneus. The grooves, respectively termed the sulcus talus and the sulcus calcaneus, when opposed form the tarsal canal. The canal is funnel shaped with the wide portion at its lateral end. The lateral opening, the sinus tarsi, can be palpated in front of the fibular malleolus especially when the foot is markedly inverted. The canal proceeds medially and posteriorly to its medial opening just behind and above the sustantaculum talus.

The posterior joint (Fig. 8) is convex on the superior surface of the calcaneus and concave on the inferior surface of the talus. Motion at this joint is principally that of inversion and eversion (Fig. 9) with the calcaneus providing most of this motion as the talus is "locked" within

5

FIGURE 5. Motion of talus within mortice: dorsiflexion and plantar flexion. As the ankle dorsiflexes, the wider anterior portion of the talus wedges in the mortice and the fibula rises causing the interosseous ligament to become horizontal. When the mortice has been fully expanded, it prevents further dorsiflexion. On plantar flexion the narrow portion of the talus presents itself and the fibula descends. Here the fibers resume their oblique direction and the mortice decreases its width.

the ankle mortice. This motion can be tested clinically by first placing the foot in marked dorsiflexion, thus "locking" the talus, then grasping the calcaneus to elicit lateral and medial motion.

The anterior facets of the subtalar joint (Fig. 8) consist of two similar surfaces on the superior aspect of the calcaneus and the inferior aspect of the body and neck of the talus. The facets of the neck and body of the talus are convex, and those of the calcaneus are concave. This is exactly contrary to the relationship of the posterior portion of the talocalcaneal joint where the calcaneal facet is convex and the talar portion of the joint is concave.

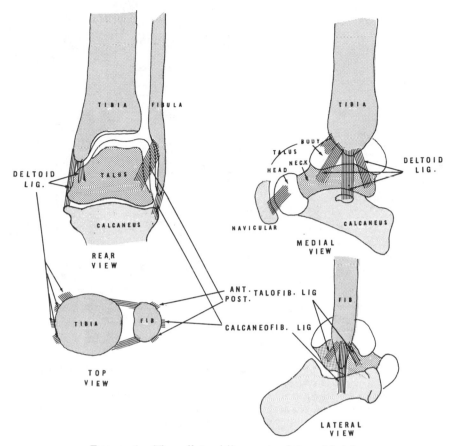

FIGURE 6. The collateral ligaments of the ankle joint.

The talonavicular joint is related to the subtalar joint and is formed by the fitting of the large convex surface of the head of the talus into the posterior concave surface of the navicular bone (Fig. 10). This joint is a part of the transverse tarsal joint.

The subtalar axis about which the calcaneus rotates in respect to the talus has a 45 degree angle to the floor and a 16 degree angle medial to a line drawn through the second metatarsal (Fig. 11). Three types of movement occur in combination about this axis: (1) about the longitudinal axis, *inversion* which consists of elevation of the medial border and depression of the lateral border of the foot and the opposite movement of *eversion*, (2) *abduction* which is outward rotation about a vertical axis through the tibia and *adduction* which is inward rotation, and (3) *dorsiflexion* and *plantar flexion* about the transverse axis. This last movement is similar to but significantly less than the motion of the talus on the tibia.

When all of these types of subtalar motions occur simultaneously they

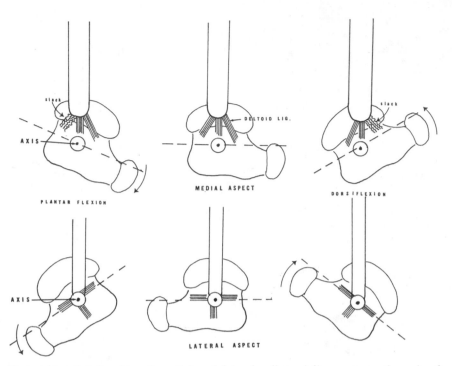

FIGURE 7. Relationship of medial and lateral collateral ligaments to the axis of ankle motion. The transverse axis of the ankle mortice transects the center of attachment of the lateral ligaments at the tip of the fibula. Plantar or dorsiflexion of the ankle does not change the length of the ligaments. The axis is eccentric to the medial deltoid ligament. During plantar flexion the posterior strands become slack and the anterior fibers taut. The opposite occurs during dorsiflexion.

result in *supination* of the foot, a combination of inversion, adduction, and plantar flexion, and *pronation* of the foot, a combination of eversion, abduction, and dorsiflexion.

The interosseous talocalcaneal ligament (Fig. 8) binds the calcaneus to the talus. It runs the length of the tarsal canal and forms a partition between the anterior and posterior portions of the talocalcaneal joints. At its fibular end there is a discrete fibrous band which connects two small tubercles opposing each other on the talus and the calcaneus. This firm band, about which some rotation can occur, is termed the ligamentum cervicis.

Because the interosseous talocalcaneal ligament runs perpendicular to the subtalar axis and because most of the ligament plus the ligamentum cervicis lies lateral to it, it tenses during inversion of the foot and is slack during eversion. This ligamentous action increases the stability of the supinated foot. The interosseous ligament can be palpated at the large

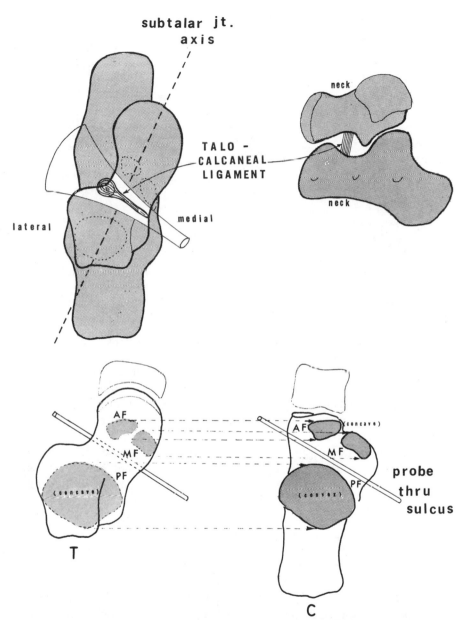

FIGURE 8. Subtalar joint (talocalcaneal joint). The talus and the calcaneus are joined by three facets. AF, anterior, MF, middle, and, PF, posterior. The sinus tarsi (tarsal canal) in its oblique course contains the talocalcaneal ligament that binds the two bones.

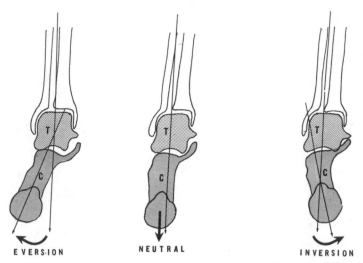

E VERS·ION   NEUTRAL   INVERSION

FIGURE 9. Motion of the subtalar (talocalcaneal) joint. The talus is fixed within the ankle mortice and has no lateral motion. The calcaneus has medial and lateral motion upon the inferior surface of the talus. The degree of inversion and eversion is restricted by the talocalcaneal ligament and the collateral ligaments of the ankle.

opening of the tarsal canal just in front of the fibular malleolus when the canal is opened by inversion.

The degree of inversion and eversion of the talocalcaneal joint is further limited by a small bony process located on the lateral inferior aspect of the body of the talus that impinges upon a similar process on the adjacent calcaneus. These processes contact upon eversion of the heel and restrict further eversion.

The transverse tarsal joint consists of the talonavicular and the calcaneocuboid joints. It has been termed the "surgeon's tarsal joint," the midtarsal joint, or Chopart's joint and is often the site of amputation of the foot.

The rounded head of the talus fits into the cupped surface of the navicular. Motion of this joint is that of rotation about an axis through the talus which slants in a forward, downward, and medial direction. The articular surface of the head of the talus is larger than the adjoining surface of the navicular which permits significant gliding at the talonavicular joint allowing inversion and eversion of the foot.

The calcaneocuboid joint has a limited range of motion permitting some abduction and adduction. When the axis of the talonavicular joint runs parallel to the axis of the calcaneocuboid joint, total motion is free and the foot is unstable. This is the situation in the pronated foot. When the two axes diverge, as they do in the supinated foot, motion of the transverse tarsal joint is restricted and the foot is more stable. This function plus the tautness of the interosseous ligament is the reason for the foot being most stable in the supinated position.

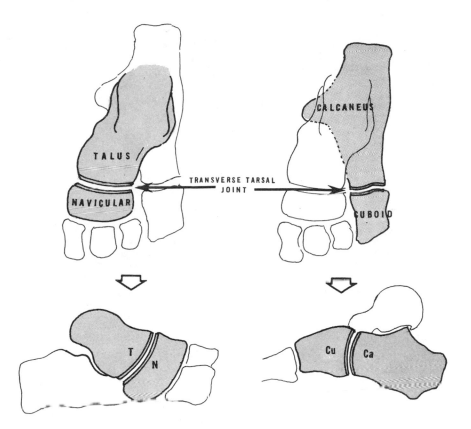

FIGURE 10.   Transverse tarsal joint.

The tarsal joints distal to the subtalar joint produce the elasticity of the foot that permits accommodation to the uneven surfaces upon which man walks. The modern firm inflexible shoe markedly restricts this motion.

The middle functional segment (Fig. 1) consists of five tarsal bones: the navicular, the cuboid, and the three cuneiforms. A rigid transverse arch held together by the interosseous ligaments is formed by the three cuneiform bones and the cuboid, the middle cuneiform being the keystone (Fig. 12).

The anterior margin of the middle segment does not present a straight border to the bases of the metatarsal bones. The second cuneiform is set back forming an indentation into which the base of the second metatarsal is firmly wedged. Being seated between the first and third cuneiforms, the second metatarsal moves only in plantar flexion and dorsiflexion articulating at its base with the first and third cuneiform.

The bases of the third, fourth, and fifth metatarsals are obliquely shaped permitting a rotatory motion of the third upon the second, the fourth upon

FIGURE 11. The subtalar axis. Movement about the subtalar axis consists of supination and pronation of the foot. The axis forms a 45 degree angle with the ground and a 16 degree angle medial to a longitudinal line drawn through the second metatarsal.

the third, and the fifth around the fourth. The fifth metatarsal, contacting only the base of the fourth and the cuboid, moves through the greatest arc. This rotatory motion increases the transverse arch and thus "cups" the sole of the foot. The base of the fifth metatarsal protrudes laterally to form a sulcus through which runs the tendon of the peroneus longus muscle.

The first metatarsal is the thickest and the shortest of the metatarsals. It has a kidney-shaped base which permits not only dorsal and plantar flexion but also rotation about an arc around the base of the second meta-

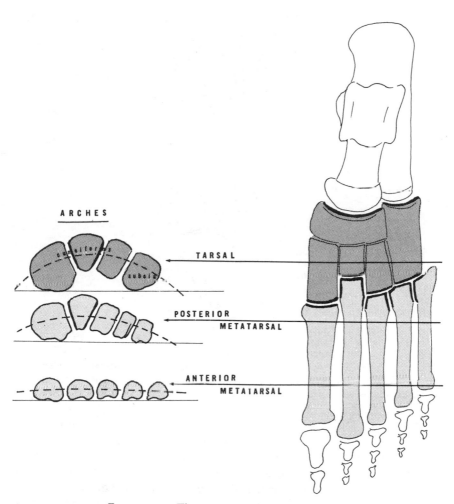

ARCHES

TARSAL

POSTERIOR
METATARSAL

ANTERIOR
METATARSAL

FIGURE 12. The transverse arches of the foot.

tarsal. The base is also shaped to permit gliding motion upon the surface of the first cuneiform. The anterior tibial and peroneus longus tendons attach upon the plantar surface of the first metatarsal (Fig. 13).

Under the head of the first metatarsal there are two small facets for the articulation of the two sesamoid bones. These sesamoid bones, erroneously called "accessory" bones, are incorporated into the tendons of the flexor hallucis brevis and act as fulcrum in the function of the tendon. They also bear body weight.

The forward projected length of the metatarsals follows a sequence of 2>3>1>4>5. The second metatarsal head protrudes the farthest with the first metatarsal being shorter than the third (Fig. 14). Excessive

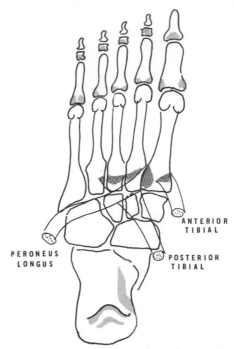

ANTERIOR
TIBIAL

PERONEUS
LONGUS

POSTERIOR
TIBIAL

FIGURE 13. Tendons that attach to the base of the first metatarsal. Viewed from the plantar surface the anterior tibial tendon attaches to the medial aspect and the peroneus longus tendon to the lateral aspect of the base of the first metatarsal.

shortening of the first metatarsal may have pathological significance as it causes the second metatarsal head to bear excessive weight.

The phalanges articulate in a gliding manner upon the large convex articular surfaces of the metatarsal heads. These surfaces extend from the plantar surface of the metatarsal heads onto the dorsum of the heads thus permitting excessive dorsiflexion of the toes. There are two phalanges in the first (big) toe (hallux) and three in all the other toes. For proper range of motion, they should be in straight alignment and the capsules and tendons sufficiently flexible to allow full flexion and extension. In every step of walking the big toe dorsiflexes; in a mile it dorsiflexes approximately 900 times. Improper alignment or lack of flexibility can traumatize the hallux joint.

Contrary to the relative forward projection of the metatarsal bones (2>3>1>4>5), the phalanges follow a sequence of 1>2>3>4>5. The first toe projects the farthest forward with the other toes gradually decreasing until the fifth toe (Fig. 14).

The tendinous action upon the phalanges of the first toe differs from all the others. Because the big toe has only two phalanges, flexor action causes the distal phalanx to "press" against the ground. There is little

14

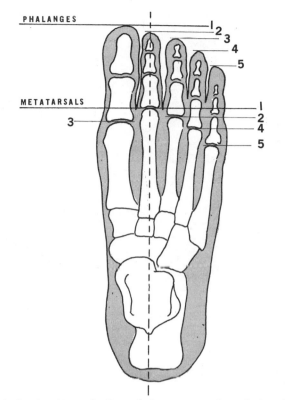

PHALANGES

METATARSALS

FIGURE 14. Relative length projection of the metatarsals and the phalanges. The relative anterior protrusion of the metatarsals follows the pattern of $2>3>1>4>5$. This makes the second metatarsal the longest and the first metatarsal the third longest. The toes have a pattern of $1>2>3>4>5$ in which the first toe protrudes farthest forward followed by each adjacent toe in regular sequence.

proximal flexion (Fig. 15). Since the other four toes each have three phalanges, the tendons cross three joints causing a "gripping" action of the toes.

MUSCLES

Muscles that originate* away from the foot and act upon the foot constitute the *extrinsic* foot muscles (Fig. 16), whereas the *intrinsic* foot

---

* The terms "origin" and "insertion" are used by most textbooks to describe muscular action with the distal appendage being free to move as the tendon and muscle direct. This description is far from accurate. During the "stance" phase of gait which constitutes 60 per cent of the walking cycle, as well as during standing, the foot is fixed to the floor causing muscular action to act upon the proximal bones. The foot is now the "origin," and the attachment of the muscles to the lower leg

FIGURE 15. Action of the flexor tendons. The tendons of the big toe cross two joints and thus act by "pressing" the distal phalanx to the floor. The sesamoid bones are incorporated into the tendons of the flexor hallucis brevis, FHB, and act to fulcrum the flexor action. The flexor tendons of the other four toes cross three joints and act to "grip" the floor. This action is performed by the flexor digitorum brevis, FDB, and longus, FDL.

muscles originate and insert within the foot itself (Fig. 17, 18, 19, and 20).

The plantar flexors of the ankle are the powerful gastrocnemius and soleus muscles. The *gastrocnemius* originates above the knee by two heads, one connected to each femoral condyle. Halfway down the leg it ends in a flat tendon, the tendo Achillis, that attaches to the posterior aspect of the calcaneus and functions to plantar flex the ankle. When the foot is weight bearing, the tendo Achillis elevates the heel from the floor. Due to the obliquity of the subtalar axis (Fig. 11), the gastroc-soleus group is also a powerful supinator at the subtalar joint when the forefoot is fixed on the floor.

The *soleus muscle* lies under the gastrocnemius and originates from the upper tibia and fibula below the knee joint. It acts upon the ankle joint but does not have ability to flex the knee as does the gastrocnemius. It ends as the deep portion of the tendo Achillis midway down the leg.

now becomes the "insertion," a reversal of the ordinary textbook designation. The opposite occurs when the foot is non-weight bearing and thus a free moving appendage. This dual role of muscular action will be discussed further under "Gait Determinants" in Chapter 3.

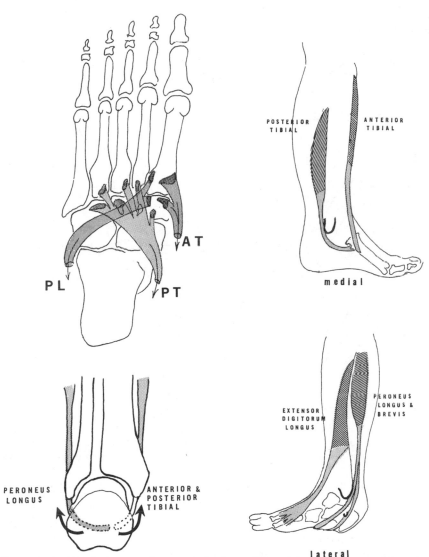

FIGURE 16.   Extrinsic musculature of the foot. The origin, direction, and insertion of the extrinsic muscles acting upon the foot are shown. The anterior tibial, AT, and the posterior tibial, PT, are medial muscles that invert the foot. The peroneus longus, PL, everts the foot. Both the posterior tibial and the peroneus longus also plantar flex the foot. The extensor digitorum and the anterior tibial dorsiflex the foot.

With the foot fixed on the ground the action of the gastroc-soleus group moves the tibia backwards, a reversed origin-insertion action. With the knee flexed the soleus is able to plantar flex the foot and ankle, whereas in the knee flexed position the gastrocnemius loses its effectiveness.

FIGURE 17. Center of gravity in two legged stance. With the person standing and balancing on both feet the feet describe an arc with the feet "toeing out" 30 degrees. The center of gravity, CG, of the body is midway between the two navicular bones.

During standing balance, with both feet planted firmly on the ground, lateral stability is maintained easily, and muscular action is needed only to prevent forward and backward sway over the center of gravity. In the average stance the feet evert to form an angle of 30 degrees, and a plumb line dropped from the sacral promontory falls midway between the feet onto a line between the navicular bones (Fig. 17). The long digital flexors (Fig. 15) create a firm pressure of the toes on the ground, and the tendons that run down the medial side of the ankle afford lateral stability by preventing eversion of the ankle.

In a relaxed stance, the plumb line passes 3 degrees in front of the talus, and the gastroc-soleus group pulls the leg back to maintain balance (Fig. 18). In relaxed erect stance no muscular action is needed anywhere in the body other than the tonic contraction of the gastroc-soleus group. The remainder of the support is ligamentous. Should the center of gravity

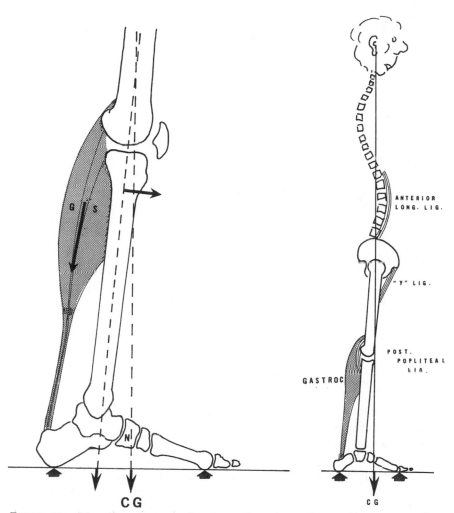

FIGURE 18. Muscular effort of relaxed two legged standing position. In standing on both feet in a relaxed manner the spine leans on the anterior longitudinal ligament, the hip on the iliofemoral "Y" ligament, and the knees extend to lean on the posterior popliteal ligaments. The gastroc-soleus must maintain tonus to pull the leg back because the center of gravity falls some 3 degrees ahead of the talus. Relaxed erect posture is principally ligamentous with only the gastroc-soleus group active. From: Cailliet, R., Low Back Pain Syndrome. F. A. Davis Co., 1962.

shift posteriorly, the anterior leg muscles, the ankle dorsiflexors, with the foot fixed on the ground, pull the leg forward.

All the tendons passing behind the malleoli are considered as plantar flexors. Medially these are the tibialis posterior, the flexor digitorum longus, and the flexor hallucis longus. Laterally the muscles consist of the peroneus longus and brevis. These groups of muscles contribute merely

19

FIGURE 19. Muscular action for lateral stability in one legged stance. As the body sways lateral to the center of gravity, CG, the medial muscles (tibialis anterior and tibialis posterior) act from the fixed foot to pull medially.

5 per cent of the total pull used to lift the heel off the ground. The big responsibility for this action belongs to the gastroc-soleus muscles.

When stance is attempted on one foot, stability is dependent upon the lateral and medial tendons acting across the ankle joint. With the foot fixed on the floor, the tendons crossing the medial half of the foot pull the leg medially and those crossing the lateral half pull laterally (Fig. 16).

If the center of gravity shifts laterally to the talus during one-leg balance, the tendons on the medial aspect of the foot pull the leg medially over the foot. These muscles are principally the *tibialis posterior* and the *tibialis anterior* (Fig. 19). This balancing adjustment requires very little muscular action. The sensory feedback from the plantar nerves initiates this coordinated muscular effort both in the specific muscle and the exact amount of contraction. Much of the sensory feedback comes from the toes which are forced to the ground, the big toe pressing and the other four toes gripping (Fig. 15). The muscular action involved in standing balance does not apply to muscular action when walking. This will be discussed in Chapter 3.

The remainder of the lower leg muscles acting upon the foot are divided into three groups: lateral, anterior, and medial. The lateral group contains the *peroneus longus* and *brevis* arising from the lateral aspect of the fibula. The longus arises higher upon the fibula and is the most superficial. Both their tendons share a common synovial sheath as they pass behind the lateral malleolus. The peroneus brevis attaches to the base of the fifth metatarsal while the peroneus longus runs deeply across the plantar surface of the foot to attach to the base of the first metatarsal and the medial cuneiform (Fig. 13). Their primary function is to evert the ankle.

The anterior group of muscles is comprised of the extensor digitorum longus, the peroneus tertius, the extensor hallucis longus, and the tibialis anterior. The tibialis anterior originates from the lateral aspect of the tibia and crosses the dorsum of the foot to insert upon the medial cuneiform and the base of the first metatarsal (Fig. 13). Its action is that of inversion and dorsiflexion of the foot.

The *extensor hallucis longus* arises from the anterior surface of the fibula and the interosseous membrane, passes across the dorsum of the foot, and inserts upon the distal phalanx of the great toe. Its action is that of extension of the hallux. It also assists to dorsiflex the ankle.

The *extensor digitorum longus* originates from the lateral condyle of the tibia and the anterior surface of the fibula and attaches by way of four tendons into the dorsal aspects of the four lateral toes. Each tendon divides at its end into a central slip that inserts upon the middle phalanx and two slips that divide and insert upon the distal phalanx. The *peroneus tertius* seems to be part of the extensor digitorum longus but attaches to the base of the fifth metatarsal bone. The extensor digitorum longus extends the toes and together with the peroneus tertius assists in dorsiflexing and everting the foot.

The medial group of lower leg muscles are the *tibialis posterior*, the *flexor digitorum longus* and *flexor hallucis longus*. Their tendons pass behind and under the medial malleolus. The tibialis posterior arises from the tibia and the fibula posteriorly and attaches by multiple fibrous extensions into most of the tarsals and medial metatarsals. Its function is inversion and plantar flexion of the foot.

The flexor hallucis longus originates somewhat laterally from the fibula and the tibia and from this posterior origin passes obliquely across the lower leg to pass under the medial malleolus and attach upon the distal phalanx of the big toe. It crosses two joints and primarily acts to press the distal phalanx to the floor (Fig. 15). The flexor digitorum longus arises from the posterior aspect of the tibia and passes behind the medial malleolus into the sole of the foot to attach to the distal phalanx of the four lateral toes. Its action is flexion of the toes in a "gripping" manner.

Inversion of the foot takes place at the subtalar and the transverse tarsal joints by means of tendons that traverse the inner border of the foot. Eversion occurs also at the subtalar joints by action of the laterally placed tendons. The peronei act most effectively as evertors when the foot is plantar flexed, and though they are mechanically situated to plantar flex the foot, they do so ineffectively. Both evertors and invertors of the ankle act as stabilizers when the foot is fixed on the floor.

The muscles of the sole of the foot, commonly called the *intrinsics* of the foot, cannot be tested individually with any clinical significance. Their major function is that of "cupping" the sole of the foot, and their innervation is from the medial and lateral plantar branches of the posterior tibial nerve. They function vitally as a source of strength to the natural longitudinal arch of the foot in conjunction with the bony architecture of the foot, the ligamentous stability, and the long muscles and their tendons which pass under the foot.

The muscles supplied by the *medial plantar nerve* (abductor hallucis, flexor digitorum brevis, flexor hallucis brevis, and the first lumbrical) function primarily to plantar flex the toes, especially the metatarsophalangeal joint of the big toe. They also stabilize the first toe phalanges at the final push-off during walking. The muscles supplied by the lateral plantar nerve maintain the arches of the foot, flex the remaining toes at the metatarsophalangeal joints, and adduct and abduct the toes. This latter function is lost in many people but the major function discernible clinically is the power of flexion at the metatarsophalangeal joints. Detailed anatomical discussion of the muscles of the sole of the foot is intentionally omitted and the reader is referred to textbooks in anatomy. The four layers of muscle are shown in Figures 20, 21, 22, and 23, and the specific innervation is summarized in Figure 24.

The *plantar fascia* is a continuation of the plantaris tendon. Its origin is upon the medial tubercle of the calcaneus from which it proceeds anteriorly and splits into five bands to attach to each digit. Each band splits at the metatarsophalangeal joint to attach to the inner and outer side of the joints and their plantar ligaments (Fig. 25). Through this split in the plantar fascia pass the long and short flexor tendons.

The medial and lateral portions of the fascia cover the abductors and short flexors or the big and little toes. There is frequently a short fibrous band that projects from the lateral aspect of the calcaneal tubercle to attach to the base of the fifth metatarsal and forms part of the lateral spring of the longitudinal arch.

NERVE SUPPLY

The nerves to the muscles of the lower leg and foot are shown in Figure 26. The *tibial nerve* is essentially a continuation of the sciatic nerve and enters the lower leg between the two heads of the gastrocnemius and passes deep to the soleus to enter the posterior compartment of the leg.

FIGURE 20. Muscles of the sole of the foot:
first layer.
Adq = Abductor digiti quinti
Ah = Abductor hallucis
Fdb = Flexor digitorum brevis

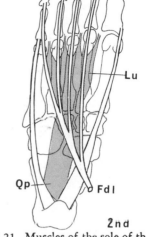

FIGURE 21. Muscles of the sole of the foot:
second layer.
Qp = Quadratus plantae
Lu = Lumbricales
Fdl = Tendon of flexor digitorum longus

FIGURE 22. Muscles of the sole of the foot:
third layer.
Aht = Adductor hallucis: transverse head
Aho = Adductor hallucis: oblique head
Fhb = Flexor hallucis brevis
Fdq = Flexor digiti quinti brevis

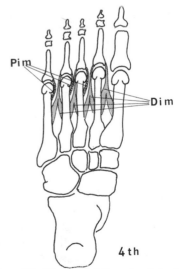

FIGURE 23. Muscles of the sole of the foot:
fourth layer.
Pim = Plantar interosseous muscles
Dim = Dorsal interosseous muscles

23

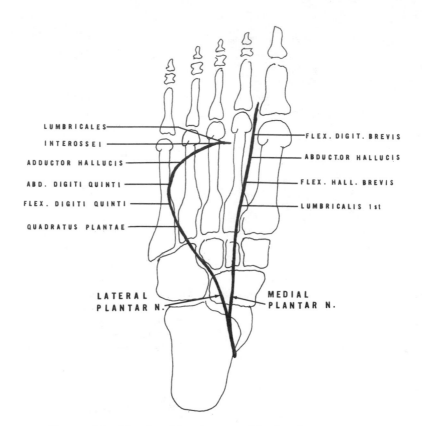

FigURE 24. Muscles of foot innervated by the plantar nerves.

The sciatic nerve ends at the upper angle of the popliteal space where it divides into the tibial and the common peroneal nerves.

The tibial nerve supplies the posterior muscles of the leg and innervates the plantar flexors of the foot. It terminates in divisions of the plantar nerves, a medial and lateral plantar branch (Fig. 26).

The *medial plantar nerve* sends cutaneous sensory branches to the plantar surface of the medial three toes and the medial aspect of the fourth toe. Its motor branches supply the abductor hallucis, flexor hallucis brevis, flexor digitorum brevis, and the first two lumbricales (Fig. 21, 22, 23, 24).

The *lateral plantar nerve* passes across the plantar surface of the foot and, after dividing into deep and superficial branches, supplies the sensation to the plantar surface of the remaining toes on the lateral aspect of the foot. It supplies the motor innervation to the quadratus plantae, flexor digiti quinti brevis, abductor digiti quinti, and the remaining plantar interosseous and lumbrical muscles.

The other division of the sciatic nerve, the *common peroneal nerve,* passes laterally out of the popliteal space. It passes behind the head of

24

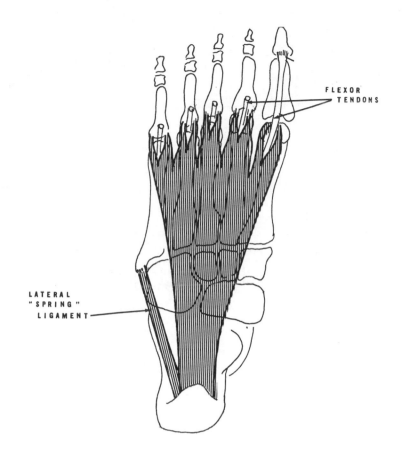

FLEXOR TENDONS

LATERAL "SPRING" LIGAMENT

FIGURE 25. Plantar fascia. The plantar fascia originates from the calcaneal tubercle. Anteriorly it splits at each metatarsophalangeal joint to permit passage of the flexor tendons. A fibrous lateral band proceeds forward to attach to the base of the fifth metatarsal which forms part of the lateral "spring" ligament.

the fibula beneath the deep fascia and winds around the lateral aspect of the fibular neck. The common peroneal nerve supplies no musculature. It merely supplies small nerve twigs to the knee joint and ultimately divides into the superficial and deep peroneal nerves (Fig. 26). The superficial peroneal nerve descends the leg in front of the fibula. It supplies the evertor muscles of the foot. The sensory area of the superficial peroneal nerve is the lateral aspect of the lower leg and the dorsum of the foot. The deep peroneal nerve proceeds to the interosseous membrane between the tibia and fibula and descends the leg supplying the dorsiflexors of the foot and ends supplying the extensor digitorum brevis. It supplies a small area of sensation between the first two toes on the dorsum of the foot. Both the deep and the superficial peroneal nerves terminate in sensory

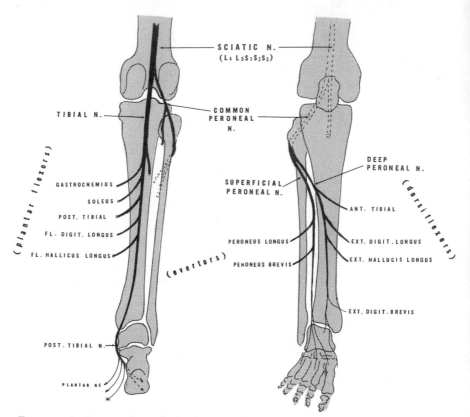

FIGURE 26. Innervation of the leg and foot. The sciatic nerve divides at the popliteal angle to form the tibial nerve and the common peroneal nerve.

branches that supply the dorsum of the foot and anterolateral aspect of the leg (Fig. 27).

BLOOD SUPPLY

The *popliteal artery* is a direct continuation of the femoral artery which passes into the posterior popliteal quadrant and divides into the anterior and posterior tibial arteries going below the knee. The posterior tibial artery follows the same course as the tibial nerve (Fig. 26) and supplies the posterior muscles of the leg. Upon reaching the medial malleolus, it passes to the plantar surface of the foot to divide into the medial and lateral plantar arteries. Below the bifurcation of the popliteal artery, the popliteal artery branches off laterally, passes across the interosseous membrane, and descends the lateral aspect of the leg to supply the lateral muscles. It ends as the *lateral calcaneal artery*.

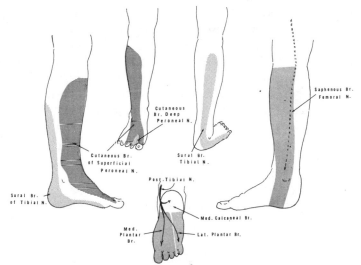

FIGURE 27. Sensory patterns of peripheral nerves of the leg.

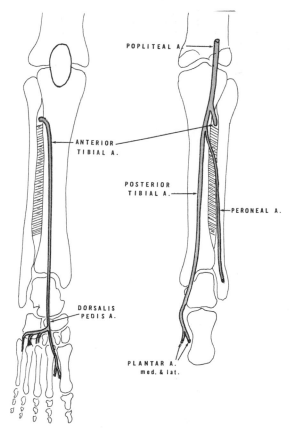

FIGURE 28. Arterial supply of the leg and foot.

Below the popliteal quadrant the popliteal bifurcation gives rise to the *anterior tibial artery* which passes anteriorly between the tibia (Fig. 28) and fibula, across the upper margin of the interosseous membrane, then courses down the anterior surface of the membrane. It supplies the muscles of the anterior compartment of the leg and reaches the dorsum of the foot as the *dorsalis pedis artery*. The terminal branches form the *dorsal metatarsal arteries* and *dorsal digital arteries*. They communicate with the plantar distal branches of the plantar arteries.

BIBLIOGRAPHY

Grant, J. C. Boileau: A Method of Anatomy, ed. 5. The Williams & Wilkins Co., Baltimore, 1952.

Gray, H.: Anatomy of the Human Body, edited by C. M. Goss. Lea & Febiger, Philadelphia, 1966.

Hicks, J. H.: Axis Rotation at Ankle Joint. J. Anat. 86:1. 1952.

Hicks, J. H.: Mechanics of the Foot. J. Anat. 87:345, 1953.

Haymaker, W., and Woodhall, B.: Peripheral Nerve Injuries: Principles of Diagnosis, ed. 2. W. B. Saunders Co., Philadelphia, 1953.

Hollinshead, W. H.: Functional Anatomy of the Limbs and Back. W. B. Saunders Co., Philadelphia, 1952.

Jones, F. W.: Talocalcaneal Articulation. Lancet. 2:241, 1944.

Jones, F. Wood: Structures and Function as Seen in the Foot, ed. 2. Bailliere, Tindall, and Cox, London, 1949.

Kaplan, E.: Some Principles of Anatomy and Kinesiology in Stabilizing Operations of the Foot. Clin. Orthop. 34: 7, 1964.

Lake, N. C.: The Foot, ed. 3. Bailliere, Tindall, and Cox, London, 1943.

Lapidus, P. W.: Kinesiology and Mechanical Anatomy of the Tarsal Joints. Clin. Orthop. 30: 20, 1963.

Mennell, J.: The Science and Art of Joint Manipulation, ed. 2. J. & A. Churchill Ltd., London, 1949.

Rubin, G., and Witten, M.: The Talar Tilt Angle and the Fibular Collateral Ligament. J. Bone Joint Surg. 42A:311, March 1960.

CHAPTER 2

Examination of the Foot

The foot is one of the few segments of human anatomy that can be fully examined. All the significant functional elements of the foot are readily accessible either visually, by palpation, or by passive motion by the examiner.

Pain, difficulty in walking, and awkwardness of gait are the foot problems that usually cause the patient to consult a physician. Foot pain may occur during standing or walking. The former may be considered the *static* foot and the latter the *kinetic*. Therefore, the foot must be examined in relaxation, weight bearing, and during walking. The examiner must develop a meaningful pattern and sequence of examination to determine the cause of pain or dysfunction. Each of the criteria of the *normal foot* must be individually sought, and any deviation from normal and its significance must be recognized and appreciated.

The *normal foot* conforms to the following criteria: (a) pain free, (b) normal muscle balance, (c) absence of contracture, (d) a central heel, (e) straight and mobile toes, and (f) three sites of weight bearing while standing and during the stance phase of walking.

HISTORY

The first criterion (a) is subjective and is revealed by the patient's history. The remaining criteria are objective and are elicited by the examination.

If pain is the presenting complaint, the patient indicates the site of pain and relates its occurrence to a certain position, motion, or activity. The site of pain denotes the anatomical site of the disorder, and the examination reveals the cause.

If the complaint is an awkward, fatiguing, or cosmetically unpleasant gait, an exact description of the gait is elicited from the patient or companion. The examiner then witnesses and interprets the gait in question.

EXAMINATION OF THE SHOE

The patient's shoes are also examined as deformities of the heel, sole, or body of the shoe have diagnostic significance. The normal foot with normal gait should wear down the heel on its outer side. This generally indicates that the calcaneus is in the neutral position with the heel centrally placed and the foot slightly inverted and also implies a good heel-toe gait. The everted foot distorts the counter (Fig. 29) and the quarter and wears the heel on its inner border. A "drop foot" due to muscular weakness scuffs the toe of the shoe. The equinovarus of spastic paralysis may also cause abnormal wear of the shoe at the toe and outer border of the sole.

The deformed vamp may reveal anatomical abnormalities of the foot. Distortions here may be caused by tightness over hammer toes or hallux valgus with bunion formation. The worn areas of the sole indicate the position of the metatarsal heads (Fig. 30).

RANGE OF MOTION

Ankle

The major ranges of motion are tested during the examination of the bare foot. Ankle plantar flexion and dorsiflexion are tested both with the knee straight and with the knee bent. When the knee is straight, the gastrocnemius muscle which originates above the knee and crosses the joint is stretched. Flexing the knee eliminates the action of the gastrocnemius and permits greater motion of the ankle joint (Fig. 31). Unin-

FIGURE 29.   Components of the shoe.

"WEAR" MARK of
METATARSAL
HEADS

FIGURE 30. Examination of the sole of the shoe.

hibited ankle motion allows 20 degree dorsiflexion and 50 degree plantar flexion from the neutral position.

The range of motion at the ankle must be judged from the excursion of the hind foot rather than the forefoot so that movements in the longitudinal arch are not mistaken for ankle movements (Fig. 32). Limitation of motion at the ankle joint may indicate joint or ligamentous abnormalities or gastroc-soleus contractures.

Subtalar Joint

The subtalar and transverse tarsal joints usually work together combining the movements of inversion and eversion; however, it is clinically possible to isolate the motion of each joint. The subtalar motion is tested by holding the lower leg firmly with one hand and holding the calcaneus in the other while keeping the ankle dorsiflexed. The dorsiflexed ankle position fixes the talus firmly in the ankle mortice and prevents lateral motion. As the patient tries to invert and evert the foot the motion of the heel from side to side can be palpated. This motion occurs at the talocalcaneal joint and is usually 20 degrees to either side of midline. The calcaneus can be passively moved from side to side while the other hand firmly fixes the leg.

31

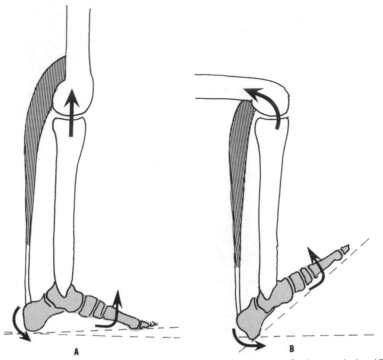

FIGURE 31. Influence of knee position on ankle plantar flexion and dorsiflexion. Because the gastrocnemius attaches above the knee joint, the ankle will not dorsiflex as much with the knee extended as it does with the knee flexed. This mechanical factor must be kept in mind when the range of ankle motion is tested clinically.

Metatarsal Joints

Midtarsal movement is tested by grasping the heel firmly with one hand while the other hand grasps the forefoot at the base of the metatarsals. Movement of the heel is manually prevented while the hand holding the forefoot pronates and supinates, adducts and abducts the forefoot. The patient inverts and everts the foot voluntarily, and the range of motion is checked passively by the examiner. The range of supination motion is greater than the range of pronation. A total pronation and supination of 40 degrees is usual.

Movements of the metatarsal bones at their proximal joints are tested individually. Because the base of the first metatarsal is kidney shaped, plantar flexion and dorsiflexion of this bone follow an arc about the base of the second metatarsal (Fig. 33) as it moves upon the first cuneiform.

The base of the second metatarsal bone is wedged between the medial and lateral cuneiforms (Fig. 12) and thus moves only in one plane, that of plantar and dorsiflexion. The third, fourth, and fifth metatarsals move in a

FIGURE 32. "False" impression of ankle dorsiflexion. The motion of the calcaneus indicates the range of motion. The forefoot may move upwards with its movement occurring at the longitudinal arch with no elongation of the gastroc-soleus group. Clinically the movement of the calcaneus indicates the extent of plantar and dorsiflexion.

plantar flexion and dorsiflexion range and arc in a rotatory manner counter to the rotation of the first metatarsal. Metatarsal motion is essentially an arcuate movement in plantar and dorsiflexion, the second metatarsal being fixed in one plane and the others moving in an arc around it. The

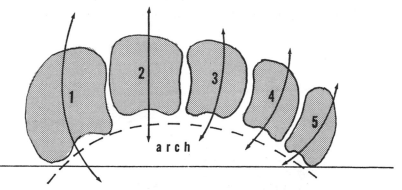

FIGURE 33. Formation of the transverse arch: movement of the individual metatarsals. The base of the second metatarsal, 2, is wedged between the medial and lateral cuneiform and can only move in one plane: dorsiflexion and plantar flexion. The first metatarsal, 1, moves in an arc about the second, 2, and the third, 3, fourth, 4, and fifth, 5, metatarsals arc in a contrary direction. Total plantar flexion of all the metatarsals about the pivot of the second forms the transverse arch.

end result of flexion is a transverse arcing of the metatarsals about the second metatarsal (Fig. 33).

The range of motion of the metarsophalangeal joint of the big toe should approach 90 degrees of dorsiflexion. Limitation of dorsiflexion to 60 degrees or less can be considered abnormal. The big toe dorsiflexes at each step in normal walking which subjects it to great stresses. Not only is it crowded by modern shoes, but it bears excessive body weight when high heels are worn.

The metarsophalangeal joint of the big toe is the site of many painful conditions such as hallux valgus, hallux rigidus, bunion, osteoarthritis, and gout and merits careful examination in the search for the cause of pain. Full dorsiflexion (extension) of the big toe exerts traction upon the plantar fascia which simultaneously elevates the longitudinal arch of the foot (Fig. 34), a fact that should be kept in mind when plantar or calcaneal pain is being investigated.

TIBIAL ALIGNMENT

After the foot has been examined in a non-weight-bearing position and each joint individually checked, it is examined with the patient sitting and the foot hanging freely. The patient should sit high enough to place his feet at the examiner's eye level. The leg is examined for alignment of the tibia with the knee and the ankle mortice. The tibial tuberosity should be directly under the patella and the dependent foot should invert slightly. "Tibial torsion" is a deviation in which the tibia is twisted on its longitudinal axis. With the patella in the midline the ankle turns inward or outward depending upon the direction of the torsion. Excess torsion is

FIGURE 34. Effect of the toes upon the longitudinal arch. Full extension of the big toe exerts traction upon the plantar fascia which causes elevation of the longitudinal arch.

34

most often found in infancy but its presence as a specific entity is questioned. It is frequently considered secondary to torsion of the femur. What appears to be a torsion of the tibia may actually be a rotation at the knee in which the tibial tubercle is medial or lateral to the patellar midline (Fig. 35). These are usually familial congenital conditions that cause a "pigeon toeing" or a "Charley Chaplin" type of gait or stance.

FEMORAL ANTEVERSION

The tibia was examined for "torsion" when the patient was seated. Now the alignment of the entire lower extremity is examined while the patient is standing. A plumb line attached to the midpoint of the patella should drop to a point between the first and second metatarsals (Fig. 35).

Deviations from normal alignment may indicate rotation of the femur and/or the tibia. Excessive rotation may be congenital or an abnormality acquired during early life. The relationship of the femoral neck to the transverse axis is called the *angle of anteversion* (Fig. 36). The transcondylar axis represents a plane passing side by side through the femur. The

FIGURE 35. Tibial and femoral torsion. The figure to the left shows the "normal" leg in which a plumb line transects the patella and touches the foot between the first and second toe. The middle picture depicts external torsion of the leg with the tibial tubercle being externally placed to the plumb line. The last picture depicts internal femoral torsion.

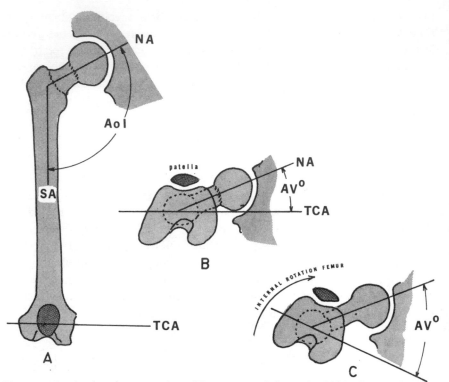

FIGURE 36. Angle of anteversion. The transcondylar axis, TCA, is a transverse line passing through the femoral condyles. An axis placed through the femoral neck, NA, forms an angle with TCA which is called the *angle of anteversion*. This is angle AV° in figure B with the femoral head viewed from above. A 15 to 25 degree angle is considered normal. In C the angle is increased due to internal rotation of the femur in relationship to the femoral neck. This is increased anteversion. Viewing the femur from anterior-posterior direction A depicts the *angle of inclination* (see Fig. 37).

normal range of anteversion is 15 to 25 degrees. An increase in this angle is an increase in anteversion and results in *internal femoral torsion*. This causes "toeing-in" during walking. Techniques for measuring femoral anteversion present radiological difficulties and have not yet been standardized.

Genu varum (bowleg) and genu valgum (knock knees) are conditions common in children. Causes must be sought when these conditions are marked or persist after infancy. Possible causes include injuries, osteomalacia, Paget's disease, or congenital variations. Congenital deviation occurs at the femoral neck in its *angle of inclination* (Fig. 37). The angle of inclination of the femoral neck is an angle formed by an axis through the femoral shaft and an axis drawn through the neck of the femur. The

FIGURE 37. Angle of inclination. The angle formed by intersecting the femoral neck angle, NA, with an axis drawn through the shaft of the femur, SA, is termed the *angle of inclination*. This angle normally varies between 116 to 140 degrees with the average being 135 degrees.

normal angle varies between 116 and 140 degrees with a greater angle forming *coxa valga* and a lesser angle *coxa vara*.

CIRCULATION

The status of the circulation is determined by noting the presence or absence of edema, dependent cyanosis, warmth or coolness of the skin, and blanching of the elevated foot. An ischemic foot will often blanch when elevated, flush when dependent, and have a thin inelastic skin lacking hair growth on the dorsum of the proximal toes. A deficient arterial blood supply is suspected when the foot becomes cyanotic on dependency and blanches on elevation.

Pitting edema noted at the end of the day and absent after a night's recumbency implies venous insufficiency. Visible varicosities enhance the diagnosis but edema, even in the presence of visible varicosities, must always raise the possibility of a systemic condition or local muscular inactivity.

Poor muscular function in the lower extremity will enhance venous stasis as surely as will prolonged dependency.

Palpation of arterial pulsations is the most significant test of the arterial circulation. The dorsalis pedis artery (Fig. 27) is felt on the dorsum of the foot between the first and second metatarsal bones (Fig. 38). The posterior tibial artery is palpable below and behind the medial malleolus of the ankle (Fig. 39). A history of claudication in which the calf cramps after walking a distance and is relieved by rest suggests arterial insufficiency. Claudication may be induced by controlled exercise in the office and will confirm the clinical history. Claudication is also suggested when walking a specified distance causes cramping or aching in the buttocks. Known as the LaReich syndrome this implies occlusive vascular disease in the more proximal circulation.

Tests to determine the adequacy of circulation include measurement of skin temperature with or without contralateral limb cooling or heating, response to intra-arterial Priscoline or other vasodilators, arteriography, and oscillometry. Such tests are in the domain of the vascular specialist, but the examiner should suspect arterial insufficiency as a possible diagnosis. Oscillometry, in which pulsations are graded by an inflated cuff, may traumatize arteriosclerotic vessels causing thrombosis and emboli and does not belong in the armamentarium of the general practitioner.

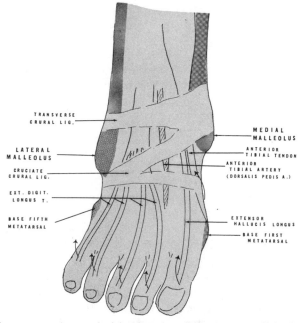

FIGURE 38. Anatomical landmarks of the dorsum of the foot.

ANTERIOR
TIBIAL

HEAD OF
TALUS

ACHILLES TENDON

POST. TIBIAL ARTERY

MEDIAL MALLEOLUS

POST. TIBIAL

FLEX. DIGIT. LONGUS

TARSAL CANAL

SUSTENTACULUM TALUS

METATARSO –
PHALANGEAL
JOINT (extension)

(flexion) SESMOID
BONES

NAVICULAR
TUBEROSITY

FIGURE 39. Anatomical landmarks of the medial aspect of the foot.

NEUROLOGICAL

A neurological examination should be performed on the non-weight bearing foot by testing the Achilles reflex, the knee reflex, the Babinski and other upper motor neuron toe signs, and by the mapping of sensory dermatome areas. Pin scratching along the foot and leg will reveal dermatome areas of hypalgesia or anesthesia corresponding to nerve root or peripheral nerve patterns (Fig. 27).

Motor Function

Motor testing is essential to the neurological examination. The sciatic nerve which arises from the L_4 to the S_2 spinal segments supplies motor function of the foot and ankle. Below the knee the sciatic nerve divides into the common peroneal nerve and the posterior tibial nerve (Fig. 26). Since each muscle group has a specific innervation the integrity of its nerve supply can be established by testing each muscle against manual resistance. The nerve supply can be further differentiated as a specific *root* or specific *peripheral nerve* establishing the site of nerve impairment.

The integrity of the tendons can also be determined during the test for muscle strength. Pain that may arise from the tendons will be localized during this phase of the examination. The anterior tibialis tendon crosses the medial aspect of the dorsum of the foot and can be visualized and palpated anterior to the medial malleolus when the foot is actively dorsiflexed and inverted. It is usually large and prominent. Ankle dorsiflexion and inversion are also assisted by the extensor hallucis longus which is primarily an extensor of the big toe. The tendon is smaller and lies on the lateral side of the anterior tibialis tendon. Its action can be eliminated by having the patient simultaneously flex the big toe while dorsiflexing the foot. The extensor hallucis longus tendon can be traced to the big toe whereas the anterior tibial tendon disappears at the medial aspect of the foot near the base of the first metatarsal.

The extensor digitorum communis tendons can be seen and felt on the lateral aspect of the dorsum of the foot as they extend to the four outer toes. They become prominent in dorsiflexion of the toes, which is their primary function, but they also assist in dorsiflexing and everting the foot. In forceful ankle dorsiflexion the anterior tibialis muscle, the extensor hallucis longus, and the extensor digitorum longus all can be seen to work simultaneously.

The plantar flexors of the foot and ankle can be tested manually but the gastroc-soleus group is so powerful that the only true test of strength and endurance is to have the patient repeatedly rise on the tiptoes of each foot individually to watch for weakness and fatigue. The extensibility of the calf muscles should be determined by passively dorsiflexing the foot with the knee extended, watching the excursion of the calcaneus, and noting any limitation of motion (Fig. 32). The degree of ankle dorsiflexion with the knee flexed establishes the elongation of the soleus muscle (Fig. 31). The markedly everted pronated foot usually has a shortened Achilles tendon and limitation of dorsiflexion; therefore, to accurately measure dorsiflexion the foot should be held in slight inversion by the examiner.

Plantar flexion of the foot and ankle is assisted by the tibialis posterior, the toe flexors, and the peroneus longus and brevis. The principal function of these muscles can be tested individually.

Inversion of the foot is initiated by the tibialis anterior muscle and the

TABLE 1—NERVE AND MUSCLE RELATIONSHIP IN DORSIFLEXION OF THE FOOT AND ANKLE

Muscle Supplied	Origin	Nerve
Tibialis anterior	L_4, L_5, S_1	deep peroneal
Extensor digitorum longus . . .	L_5, S_1	nerve branch of the
Extensor hallucis longus	L_5, S_1	common peroneal
		nerve

Muscle Supplied	Origin	Nerve
Gastrocnemius	S_1, S_2	Tibial
Soleus	L_5, S_1, S_2	
Tibialis posterior	L_5, S_1	
Flexor digitorum longus	L_5, S_1	
Flexor hallucis longus	L_5, S_1	
Peroneus longus and brevis	L_5, S_1	Superficial peroneal nerve (branch of the common peroneal nerve)

extensor hallucis longus as their tendons insert on the inner border of the forefoot. The gastrocnemius and soleus *invert* the foot. When the foot is flat on the floor and weight bearing, the Achilles tendon elevates the calcaneus. This motion occurs about the subtalar axis and causes supination of the forefoot.

The tibialis posterior is the major invertor of the foot and is innervated by the posterior tibialis nerve (Fig. 26). Its tendon can be palpated behind and below the medial malleolus when the foot is actively inverted and plantar flexed (Fig. 39).

Eversion of the foot is initiated by the extensor digitorum longus when the foot is in the neutral or dorsiflexed attitude, but in plantar flexion the peroneus longus and brevis initiate the major eversion action. The peronei receive their nerve supply from the superficial peroneal nerve (Fig. 26) and their tendons can be palpated behind and below the lateral malleolus (Fig. 40).

The four layers of the intrinsic muscles of the sole of the foot were discussed briefly in Chapter 1 (Fig. 20, 21, 22, and 23). They are innervated by the medial and lateral plantar nerves (Fig. 24) and function primarily to arch the sole of the foot in a "cupping" motion.

The gross appearance of the non-weight bearing foot is observed noting its color and skin texture. Calluses are noted and related to the underlying bone structure. Corns or calluses occur at sites of faulty weight bearing or pressures, during stance or during walking, and usually indicate improper shoe fit. Corns and calluses are found at the sites of pain and examination reveals the underlying cause.

The weight-bearing foot is now examined. A footprint gives an indication of weight-bearing points and surfaces. The longitudinal arch is checked with the patient standing. If the inner border of the foot is in contact with the floor a "flatfoot" is indicated.

FIGURE 40. Superficial anatomical landmarks of the lateral aspect of the foot.

FLATFOOT

The *flatfoot* is common and has many varied types. The flatfoot due to a fat pad under the arch is noted so frequently in infants as to be considered normal and will be discussed in Chapter 4. If the lower limb is angulated either at the femur or the tibia, the foot will pronate because the line of weight bearing falls inside the normal midline (Fig. 35) and places undue stress upon the longitudinal arch. "Knock knees" in children cause a shift in the center of gravity that may cause the foot to bear weight on its inner margin and thus flatten the foot.

Relaxed Flatfoot

A relaxed flatfoot has a good longitudinal arch which disappears upon weight bearing and usually reforms when the patient rises on his toes. This condition implies ligamentous laxity and may be congenital. It often arises in middle-aged individuals in occupations that require prolonged standing. It also occurs in people who have gained excessive weight, received inadequate exercise or experienced a period of prolonged bed rest. It need not be symptomatic nor is treatment always indicated.

In very severe flatfoot the navicular and the head of the talus are in contact with the ground and the head of the talus is very prominent. The heel and forefoot are usually everted, and the forefoot is splayed.

Rigid Flatfoot

The rigid flatfoot is a pronated foot with an inflexible depressed arch and implies soft tissue contracture, articular damage, unreduced fracture or dislocation, or bony ankylosis. A rigid flatfoot can result from fibrous contracture of the peronei muscles. X-rays may be necessary to differentiate the cause of the rigid flatfoot.

The Achilles tendon was tested for shortening during an earlier phase of the examination with the knee extended to test the gastrocnemius and the knee flexed to test the soleus (Fig. 31, 32). Achilles shortening can be tested also by having the patient lean forward against a wall keeping his knees straight and his heels in contact with the floor. Complaints of calf pain can be reproduced by this procedure (Fig. 41).

FIGURE 41. Testing tendo Achillis elongation in the erect position. The patient stands a distance from the wall and leans against it. The leg to be tested remains behind with the knee extended and the heel against the floor. The other foot is brought forward and the knee bent. The Achilles tendon is stretched as the body leans forward. The heel will rise from the floor if the Achilles is shortened, and characteristic pain can be reproduced. This movement may also be used as an exercise to stretch the heel cord.

The examination is completed by observing foot performance during walking both with and without shoes.

BIBLIOGRAPHY

Adams, J. C.: Outline of Orthopaedics, ed. 5. The Williams & Wilkins Co., Baltimore, 1964.

Bailey, H.: Demonstrations of Physical Signs in Clinical Surgery, ed. 13. The Williams & Wilkins Co., Baltimore, 1960.

Gartland, J. J.: Fundamentals of Orthopaedics. W. B. Saunders, Philadelphia, 1965.

Haymaker, W., and Woodhall, B.: Peripheral Nerve Injuries: Principles of Diagnosis. W. B. Saunders Co., Philadelphia, 1959.

Lewin, P.: The Foot and Ankle, ed. 4. Lea & Febiger, Philadelphia, 1959.

Milgram, J. E.: Office Measures for Relief of the Painful Foot. J. Bone & Joint Surg. 46:1095, 1964.

Oester, Y. T., and Mayer, J. H.: Motor Examination of Peripheral Nerve Injuries. Charles C Thomas, Springfield, Ill., 1960.

Ryder, C. T., and Crane, L.: Measuring Femoral Anteversion: The Problem and a Method. J. Bone Joint Surg. 35-A:321, 1953.

Schwartz, R. P., and Heath, A. L.: Pointed and Round-toed Shoes. J. Bone & Joint Surg. 48-A:2, 1966.

Wilson, J. N.: The Treatment of Deformities of the Foot and Toes. Brit. J. Phys. Med. 17:73 (April) 1954.

CHAPTER 3

The Walking Foot

To understand the role of the foot and ankle, all the components of man's gait must be evaluated. Observations on the mechanics of walking were recorded as far back as Aristotle and Leonardo da Vinci, and in recent decades all components of walking have been studied with great scientific precision. The search for better prosthetic devices for war amputees has placed an emphasis on the study of gait *biomechanics* in this century. Three-dimensional views of gait have been analyzed by the combined use of cameras, mirrors, and electromyography. The energy expended by individual muscles in all phases of gait is being investigated to determine their contribution.

Static deformities and pathological gaits can be better understood through a thorough knowledge of normal gait. The role of the foot and ankle must be studied within all the determinants of gait.

Locomotion is the translation of the body from one point to another. Initiation of locomotion requires an interplay between the forces of gravity, inertia, and the ground as affected by the contraction of muscles acting upon the lower extremities. Human locomotion has been compared to a wheel rolling over the ground with the legs being two of its spokes. The spoke that touches the ground constitutes the "stance" phase of walking, and the spoke that moves about the axle is the "swing" phase.

If the axis of the wheel moves in a horizontal line, a minimum of energy is expended in accordance with *Newton's law of motion* which states that "a body will continue to move in a straight line unless a contrary force impells a change." All the determinants of gait minimize the forces that tend to impede effortless motion. In essence, man attempts to keep his center of gravity moving in a straight horizontal line during locomotion.

Man's center of gravity is located just anterior to his second sacral vertebra, midway between both hip joints. Walking is initiated by inclining the body forward thus placing it ahead of its center of gravity. To regain balance, one leg must be brought forward ahead of the shifting center of gravity. The leg that remains weight bearing is the "stance" leg and must always be in contact with the ground.

The leg that moves to regain balance is the "swing" limb. The stance leg as it remains to the rear of the center of gravity helps to propel the body forward. Walking therefore can be divided into a "stance" phase, in which a leg is weight bearing, and a "swing" phase, in which the leg is moved to another point of contact. The stance phase occupies about 60 per cent of the *gait cycle,* which begins as the heel strikes the ground and ends after the swing phase has again found the same heel "striking."

GAIT DETERMINANTS

If man were to walk with his knees stiff and his pelvis moving in a straight line, his center of gravity would describe a high undulating pathway. Its highest point would occur when the stiff weight-bearing leg was vertical (mid-stance) and its lowest when one limb is fully flexed and the other extended at the hip (double stance) (Fig. 42). This type of gait would be jerky and require a great deal of energy to alternately elevate and depress the body weight at each step. Man does not walk this way but normally uses various movements of his hips, knees, ankles, and pelvis to maintain his center of gravity on a horizontally level plane. These movements are known as *determinants of gait;* together they increase efficiency, decrease energy expenditure, and make the gait more graceful.

During a complete cycle, the center of gravity is displaced twice in its vertical axis. The peak occurs during the middle of the stance phase when the weight-bearing leg is vertical and its lowest point when both legs are weight bearing with one at the position of *heel strike* and the other at *toe-off.* The undulating center of gravity may transcribe a cycle that has a vertical displacement of 2 in.

FIGURE 42. Undulant course of pelvic center in gait without determinants. The marked vertical undulations of the center of gravity occur when gait is performed with stiff knees and no lateral motion of the pelvis.

Pelvic Rotation

Decrease of the height of the vertical undulations is attempted by *pelvic rotation* in which the pelvis oscillates about an axis of the lumbar spine. Viewed from above, one side of the pelvis comes forward with the limb that is swinging forward. This movement lessens the angle between the pelvis and the thigh which also lessens the angle between the leg and the floor. The extent that the pelvis depresses during the step is also decreased (Fig. 43). The pelvis rotates approximately four degrees on each side, with a total rotation of 8 degrees, and by this rotation, the vertical undulation of the center of gravity is decreased by $\frac{3}{8}$ in.

Pelvic Tilt

Another determinant of gait is *pelvic tilt* (Fig. 44), a drop of the pelvis on the swing side. The stance leg at this point is adducted, and the swinging leg is slightly abducted (Fig. 45) and flexed at the hip and knee to clear the floor. This flexion with the simultaneous "Trendelenburg position" of the other hip decreases the vertical undulation by an additional $\frac{1}{8}$ in.

Knee Flexion during Stance Phase

The third determinant of gait is *knee flexion* during the stance phase. The knee is fully extended at heel strike which starts the stance phase for that leg. As the body moves over its center of gravity the knee flexes (Fig. 46) approximately 15 degrees until the foot is flat upon the ground. The body then passes over the foot, and the knee gradually re-extends to

FIGURE 43. Pelvic rotation: first determinant of gait. The pelvis rotates forward with the "swinging" leg thus decreasing the angle formed by the leg with the floor and at the hip joint. This rotation decreases the vertical undulations of the center of gravity of the pelvis.

FIGURE 44. Pelvic tilt: second determinant of gait. Pelvic rotation is shown in 1. As the left leg swings through, the pelvis on the left drops, 2, and the left hip and knee flex. The last figure on the right shows the right leg swinging through with the right side of the pelvis dipping and the right hip and knee flexing.

FIGURE 45. Composite of first two determinants of gait. VD shows vertical displacement from the side view. PR is pelvic rotation as the leg swings through. PT indicates pelvic tilt. The bottom figures illustrate gait from the front and show lateral shift of the pelvis combined with tilt and rotation. The weight bearing leg, W, goes into a "Trendelenburg position": adducting as the pelvis shifts over it. The swinging leg is slightly abducted. PS indicates pelvic shift and the arrows the direction of the shift.

KNEE
EXTENDED   KNEE
FLEXES   KNEE
FLEXED   KNEE
FLEXED   KNEE
EXTENDS

HEEL
STRIKE   ANKLE DORSIFLEXES   HEEL
OFF

FIGURE 46. Knee flexion during stance phase: third determinant of gait. The knee is fully extended at heel strike. As the body passes over the center of gravity the knee flexes to decrease the vertical amplitude of the pathway of the center of gravity. The knee re-extends at the end of the stance phase: the "heel off."

full extension at the end of the stance phase. This knee flexion decreases the extent of pelvic undulation by an additional $\frac{1}{8}$ in.

Knee-Ankle Relationship

The fourth determinant upon gait is a combined *motion of the knee and ankle*. This knee action, although similar to the third determinant, is different in relating principally to ankle motion in its influence upon the pathway of pelvic undulation. At heel strike the ankle is dorsiflexed to about 90 degrees and gradually plantar flexes to become flat on the ground as the body approaches the center of gravity. This rotation occurs about the ankle joint. As the ankle joint passes over the weight-bearing heel, two small arcs of motion occur which the knee, by slight flexion, smooths out (Fig. 47).

Pelvic Shift

A last determinant is *pelvic shift* in which the pelvis moves laterally to maintain body balance as one leg is lifted from the ground. As the pelvis shifts, the weight-bearing limb adducts (Fig. 45). This sway from side to side smooths the pelvic movement as well as maintaining balance.

The determinants of pelvic rotation, pelvic tilting, knee and ankle flexion, and pelvic shift all aim to decrease the amplitude of vertical displacement of the pelvis and to decrease the degree of undulation. Both of these decrease the energy required to raise and lower the body during walking.

A flattened pathway in the vertical displacement increases the *relative* length of the lower extremity thus increasing the length of the stride without increasing the degree of hip flexion and extension. As the speed of

ANKLE ARCS

FIGURE 47. Foot and ankle relationship: fourth determinant of gait. At the heel strike the ankle is dorsiflexed 90 degrees. The level of the ankle rises slightly as the foot goes forward into the "flatfoot stance" phase. This is followed by the ankle again dorsiflexing as the leg passes over the foot. At push-off the heel rises giving a second small upward undulation. These two small undulations at the ankle are *smoothed out* by simultaneous knee flexions.

locomotion is dependent upon the length of the stride rather than an increase in cadence, the determinants of gait improve forward velocity without increasing gait cadence and thus further conserve energy.

The above determinants concern motion of the lower extremity in a sagittal plane. During locomotion there is a transverse rotation of the lower extremity which also facilitates gait. In addition to the rotation of the pelvis, which has been mentioned, the thigh, leg, and ankle also rotate about the longitudinal axis.

As the limb begins its swing phase the femur begins to rotate internally, and simultaneously the tibia rotates internally upon the femur. This rotation continues past heel strike into the stance phase and ends when the foot is fully flat upon the ground. It is at this point that the opposite leg begins its swing phase and its internal rotation.

Once the foot is flat, derotation begins as the pelvis passes over the fixed weight-bearing foot. Simultaneously the stance hip and tibia gradually rotate externally. Any rotation in the foot must occur at the subtalar joint because the foot is fixed to the floor and no lateral motion is permitted at the ankle mortice.

The average angle of "toe-out" of the weight-bearing foot to the plane of forward progression is usually 6 to 7 degrees (Fig. 48). A greater degree of toeing out occurs in the aged and improves balance. In faster walking, stability is less of a problem and toeing out decreases to the point of being totally eliminated.

FIGURE 48. Outward angulation of the feet during walking. A "toe-out" angle of 6 to 7 degrees is usual but increases with aging. Faster walking decreases the toe-out to 0 degrees. Length of stride is measured from stance of the foot to the next stance of the same foot.

MUSCULAR ACTION

Locomotion depends upon muscles as movers, stabilizers, and decelerators. Muscles of the lower extremity may act across one or two joints. They may move a free segment of the extremity or act from a fixed segment.

Walking can begin with relaxation of the gastroc-soleus group to permit a forward inclination of the body ahead of the center of gravity (Fig. 18). With this shift forward, the supporting foot becomes the *propulsive* foot. The weight-bearing portion of the foot shifts from the heel, along the lateral side of the foot and across the metatarsal heads towards the pad of the big toe (Fig. 49). The big toe presses the ground stabilizing the foot and aiding in the push-off.

Major muscular activity begins during the last 10 degrees of the swing phase and ends after the first 10 degrees of the stance phase. From the activity occurring at the *end of the swing phase,* it is apparent that muscular activity decelerates the limb rather than combating gravity. After heel strike, the body is "pulled forward" over the anchored foot. The calf muscles, during the stance phase, act almost exclusively to decelerate the leg as it passes over the foot (Fig. 50). Sixty per cent of energy expended is used for deceleration rather than propulsion against gravity.

Muscular activity during gait is depicted in Figures 50 and 51. The erector spinae muscles raise the pelvis, and the glutei stabilize the hip during lateral pelvic shifting. The hip flexors initiate the swing phase, but the impetus of the swinging limb is delivered by the pendular extension of the leg upon the thigh. The quadriceps, which acts across two joints, flexes the hip while simultaneously extending the knee when the foot is free. It is during the "swing through" that the thigh and leg rotate inwardly.

Early in the swing phase the hamstring muscles flex the knee if a faster cadence is needed. At the end of the swing phase (Fig. 51) the

Toe
Off

Heel
Strike

FIGURE 49. Path of weight bearing of the foot during walking. Weight bearing begins at the heel (*heel strike*) and proceeds along the lateral border of the foot towards the metatarsal heads with the major propulsive thrust by the distal phalanx of the big toe (*toe-off*).

hamstring muscles brake the swinging lower limb to minimize the impact of knee extension.

The pretibial group of muscles is active throughout the entire swing phase to raise the toes to clear the floor. Immediately after heel strike the ankle dorsiflexors brake the plantar motion of the foot to prevent a forceful foot "slap" (Fig. 51 and 52).

The plantar flexors remain active during the middle and last portion of the stance phase. As the heel leaves the ground the plantar flexors cease all activity. Throughout most of the stance phase, as the leg passes over the foot, the ankle is dorsiflexing upon the tibia. During this dorsiflexion the pretibial muscles are inactive and the plantar flexors are contracting. This indicates that dorsiflexion of the ankle is achieved mechanically and the gastroc group is used for deceleration (Fig. 51, 52, and 53).

Shortly after heel strike, when the foot has become flat against the ground, the lower limb begins to rotate externally. The foot is now fixed on the ground so rotation of the leg and foot occurs at the subtalar joint and causes the foot to supinate (Fig. 54). This subtalar rotation aligns

FIGURE 50. Muscular activity of normal walking. The various muscular groups are related to the hip, knee, and ankle motion throughout the various aspects of the gait

FIGURE 51. Muscular activity of the lower extremity during normal gait. The muscular activity as viewed in the right leg is shown through a complete stride cycle.

FIGURE 52. Muscular activity of the leg and ankle during normal gait. This duplicates Figure 51 but concentrates upon the leg, ankle, and foot during gait from toe-off through a full stride.

54

FIGURE 53. Ankle dorsiflexion during stance phase of gait. The ankle dorsiflexes during stance phase by mechanical forces. As the leg passes over the foot the ankle is dorsiflexed *without* action of the dorsiflexor muscles. The gastroc group is active throughout this action and acts to *decelerate* the forward motion of the body. The floor applies a *shear stress* to the foot during this action.

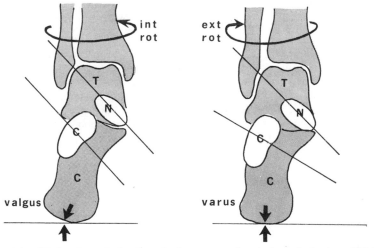

FIGURE 54. Supination of the foot during external rotation of the leg. With the foot weight bearing during stance phase, external rotation of the leg causes the foot to rotate at the subtalar joint and *supinate* the foot. The leg begins to externally rotate during walking when the foot is fully flat against the floor. The supinated position places the calcaneus into more varus and thus places the Achilles tendon in a more direct alignment with the leg.

the Achilles tendon more centrally and thus gives the plantar flexors more efficiency and the foot more stability.

The walking foot can be better understood when studied in relationship to the total biomechanics of the lower limb during gait.

BIBLIOGRAPHY

Basmajian, J. V.: Man's Posture. Arch. Phys. Med. 46:26, Jan. 1965.

Basmajian, J. V., and Stecko, G.: The Roles of Muscles in Arch Support of the Foot. J. Bone Joint Surg. 45-A:1184, 1963.

Brantingham, C. R., Egge, A. S., and Beekman, B. E.: The Effect of Artificially Varied Surface on Ambulatory Rehabilitation with Preliminary EMG Evaluation of Certain Muscles Involved. Presented at APA Annual Meeting, Los Angeles, August 1963.

Levens, A. S.., Inman, V. T., and Blosser, J. A.: Transverse Rotation of the Segments of the Lower Extremity in Locomotion. J. Bone Joint Surg. 30-A:849, 1948.

Liberson, W. T.: Biomechanics of Gait: A Method of Study. Arch. Phys. Med. 46:37, Jan. 1965.

MacConaill, M. A.: The Postural Mechanism of the Human Foot. Proc. Roy. Irish Acad. 1B:265, May 1945.

Mann, R., and Inmann, V. T.: Phasic Activity of Intrinsic Muscles of the Foot. J. Bone Joint Surg. 46-A:469, 1964.

Morton, D. J.: Human Locomotion and Body Form, A Study of Gravity and Man. Williams & Wilkins Co., Baltimore, 1952.

Murray, M. P., Drought, A. B., and Kory, R. C.: Walking Patterns of Normal Men. J. Bone Joint Surg. 46-A:335, 1964.

Murray, M. P., et al.: Comparison of Free and Fast Speed Walking Patterns of Normal Men. Amer. J. Phys. Med. 45:8, Feb. 1966.

Saunder, J. B. de C. M., Inmann, V. T., and Eberhart, H. D.: The Major Determinants in Normal and Pathological Gait. J. Bone Joint Surg. 35-A:543, 1953.

Steindler, A.: Kinesiology of the Human Body. Charles C Thomas, Springfield, Ill., 1955.

Sutherland, D. H.: An Electromyographic Study of the Plantar Flexors of the Ankle in Normal Walking on the Level. J. Bone Joint Surg. 48-A:66.

Wright, D. G., Desai, S. M., and Henderson, W. H.: Action of the Subtalar and Ankle Joint Complex during the Stance Phase of Walking. Biomechanics Laboratory, University of California, San Francisco, No. 38, June 1962.

CHAPTER 4

The Foot in Childhood

Many common foot problems seen at birth and during early childhood, if recognized and treated early, may respond to conservative treatment. Such abnormalities are more common than the literature indicates. In most cases the causative factors are more conjectural than scientific but if the mechanism causing the abnormality is recognized, appropriate corrective treatment may cure or at least minimize the deformity.

CLASSIFICATION OF FOOT DEFORMITIES

Foot deformities are generally classified into four positions: (1) *equinus* in which the heel is elevated and the foot is plantar flexed, (2) *calcaneus* in which the foot is dorsiflexed and the heel relatively depressed, (3) *varus* * in which the foot is inverted and adducted, and (4) *valgus* * in which the foot assumes a position of eversion and abduction. Deformities

---

* There is considerable confusion in the terminology used to describe position and movement of the foot.

Varus implies that the distal member of an extremity is bent *towards* the midline. The apex of the angle formed by the longitudinal axes of the component bones points away from the midline. The heel is rotated inward on its longitudinal axis or is inverted (Gartland).

Valgus means bent or turned *from* the midline. The apex of the angle formed by the longitudinal axes of the component bones points *towards* the midline. The heel in valgus is everted or rotated outwards on its longitudinal axis (Gartland).

Movement about an axis passing transversely through the foot is *dorsiflexion-plantar flexion*. Movement about a vertical axis is *abduction-adduction* and about a longitudinal axis *inversion-eversion*.

Inversion implies elevation of the inner border of the foot and *eversion* elevation of the outer border. Adduction-abduction occurs chiefly at the tarsometatarsal joints. Inversion and adduction combine to constitute *supination* and also varus of the forefoot, whereas eversion and abduction cause *pronation* or valgus of the foot.

MacConaill views the foot as a "twisted osteo-fibrous plate" by which the intrauterine position of the lower limb is in pronation and any lessening of the foot torsion is supination. The foot is thus supinated when it has been "untwisted."

may consist of just one of the above positions, but the majority are combinations in which equinus is associated with varus or valgus, or calcaneus with varus or valgus (Fig. 55).

ETIOLOGICAL CONCEPTS

The majority of foot deformities noted in infants are flatfoot and equino-varus deformities. Valgus, varus, equinus, and calcaneus abnormalities

(RIGHT FOOT)

FIGURE 55. Terminology of foot abnormalities or positions.

comprise the remainder. These abnormalities are considered to be congenital, acquired, or a residual of neurological abnormalities.

Delay or arrested derotation of the intrauterine position is one of the intriguing concepts of the causation of the abnormal foot. About the third month of intrauterine existence the fetus has its thighs flexed, abducted, and outwardly rotated with its legs crossed. The feet are plantar flexed and adducted with the plantar surfaces held against its own abdomen (Fig. 56). As the fetus develops, the thighs derotate inwardly and the feet gradually turn out to become placed against the uterine wall. If, for some reason, derotation of the feet is arrested, the child is born with the feet still plantar flexed and inverted in the equinovarus position.

There are instances in which the newborn has a postural attitude with one leg internally rotated and the other externally rotated. This birth posture is termed "windblown hips," an analogy to a sailor walking against the wind. This attitude frequently continues after birth because the child sleeps in this position.

Faulty positions of the foot may persist because of contracture of the leg muscles. In the equinus foot the plantar flexors are contracted, the evertors in the valgus foot, and the anterior dorsiflexors in the calcaneus foot. When several components of deformity exist there may be several combinations of contracture. If the abnormal position is not corrected in early childhood, the bones of the foot become structurally deformed, and correction by conservative means becomes less feasible.

FETAL POSITION

PRONE
SLEEPING
POSITION

A

B

FIGURE 56. Fetal position and sleeping posture. A depicts the fetal position with the hips flexed, abducted, and rotated outwardly. The feet are usually plantar flexed and adducted with plantar surface against the abdomen. The sleeping position, B, will maintain the newborn position. In this illustration both feet are abducted. The foot position varies with the immediate postpartum position.

At birth the foot consists of as much soft tissue as bone. X-ray of the foot shows only the diaphysis of the phalanges and the metatarsals and the nuclei of the calcaneus and talus (Fig. 57). Only the calcaneus, talus, and occasionally the cuboid are ossified at birth; the remainder of the bones are still cartilage. Growth continues from infancy through adolescence and Figure 58 shows the ages at which the centers of ossification appear and fuse. During this period of growth, structural changes in the foot may be caused by abnormal stresses. By the time it is full-grown, the foot is 90 per cent bone.

FOOT POSTURES OF THE NEWBORN

The conditions of equinus or calcaneus with either varus or valgus should be recognized early. Manual testing will determine whether the foot is sufficiently flexible to permit correction of the deformity. If the foot is flexible enough and the deformity easily altered, stretching of the soft tissues is begun immediately. The abnormality is demonstrated to the parents, and the tissue-stretching exercises taught so the child can receive the stretching several times a day. The specific exercises must be carefully prescribed, explained, and demonstrated to the parents and their performance observed for accuracy.

The forefoot may be in adduction or abduction and in mild supination

FIGURE 57. X-ray of foot in the newborn. In the newborn only the diaphyses of the phalanges and metatarsals along with the nuclei of the talus and calcaneus are visible.

OSSIFIED   FUSED

2–4 yrs ——— 18 yrs (11–22)

6 mo–3 yrs ——— 18 yrs (11-22)

2 yrs

AT BIRTH

2 yrs
2 ½ yrs
3–6 mo —— 14–21 yrs

3 yrs

AT BIRTH

5–12 yrs ———— 12 – 20 yrs

6 mo ——→ **TIBIA** ←—— 16–18 yrs

I yr ——→ **FIBULA** ←—— 16–18 yrs

FIGURE 58. Age of appearance and age of closure of the ossification centers of the foot.

or pronation. The forefoot can be moved in either direction with the other hand holding the calcaneus firmly. This maneuver tests the flexibility of the forefoot and also becomes a manner of treating any existing inflexibility. Once established as pertinent the movement is taught to the parents. If a tight Achilles tendon is discovered, this too can be stretched by the parents. They must be made aware that elevation of the forefoot does not necessarily stretch the Achilles tendon (Fig. 32). Only when the calcaneus is "pulled down" does the heel cord get stretched. The foot that is pronated (everted) usually has a shortened Achilles tendon, and to be stretched properly the foot must be inverted during the stretching exercises.

The calcaneus deformity (Fig. 55) may reveal contracture of the dorsiflexors and the toe extensors. These can be stretched by grasping the leg and gradually, firmly, and repeatedly forcing the foot into plantar flexion. The toes can be flexed simultaneously thus stretching the toe extensors.

If the deformed foot does not become more flexible and appear more nearly normal after four to six weeks of daily passive stretching, mechanical devices are indicated. Because soft-tissue changes cause and maintain the foot deformity, gradual stretching of the foot into a more physiological position can be achieved by plaster casting or by bracing. The attempt is always made to *overcorrect* the deformity so that when the tissues are released they will return with the foot to the normal position and not a partially deformed posture. Plaster casting is more satisfactory than bracing because it is skintight and by proper molding can correct the specific portion of the foot desired. Also, plaster is obviously less expensive than bracing.

The newly acquired position of overcorrection is held for one to four weeks by maintaining the cast or by bivalving the cast and applying it for varying portions of the day with interspersed exercises. Exercises must be resumed when the cast is ultimately removed. If the foot is large enough to be fitted with a "corrective" shoe, the correction can thus be maintained. The term "corrective" is questioned because no shoe corrects a deformity; it merely holds the correction gained by other means.

PRONATED FOOT

The infant foot is and appears to be *flat*. No longitudinal arch is visible, and the arch that does exist is masked by a fat pad on the sole of the foot. The navicular and cuneiform that form the apex of the longitudinal arch are still in the cartilaginous stage and are soft and compressible. The muscles and ligaments are not well developed. The foot at this stage is not ready for weight bearing. The age of two years is probably the earliest that walking is advisable. The child may be allowed to walk before this but should not be forced to do so.

The pronated foot is so common in childhood that it can be considered "normal." Excessive pronation may be considered abnormal and frequently causes parental concern. The severity of pronation can be roughly graded as mild or first degree, second degree, or third degree. Mild first-degree pronation places the weight-bearing line along the medial border of the foot with some longitudinal arch visible. Second-degree pronation changes the contour of the foot with depression of the longitudinal arch and prominence of the navicular bone. Third-degree pronation reveals a totally "flat" foot with no longitudinal arch and a footprint that reveals no indentation along the inner border. These gradings of pronation are arbitrary and contribute little to the choice of treatment or the prognosis nor do they necessarily correlate with the severity of the symptoms.

Congenital Flatfoot

The congenital flatfoot is relatively rare but when present is more severe than the acquired flatfoot (Fig. 59). In the flexible congenital flatfoot, the position is one of calcaneovalgus with the foot folded laterally upon itself. It can be brought downward with relative ease and can be so maintained until muscular action and weight bearing develop. It is maintained by daily exercising and a shoe that holds the foot in the corrected position or a plaster cast that is bivalved and worn for varying periods.

Rigid Flatfoot

The rigid flatfoot is more difficult to treat. In this condition the heel is firmly held in a marked valgus position and the forefoot in marked eversion. There is almost a reversal of the longitudinal arch which appears convex rather than concave and bulges at its midpoint. X-ray reveals that the talus faces medially and downward, and the navicular rests on the superior surface of the neck of the talus rather than in front of its head.

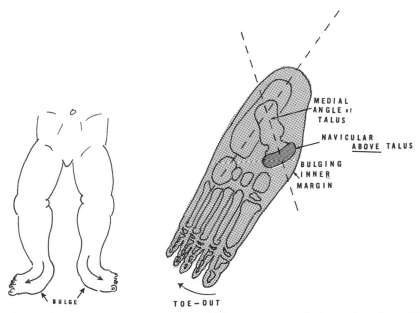

FIGURE 59. Congenital flatfoot. Congenital flatfoot is a calcaneo-valgus foot. The heel is in valgus and the talus points medially towards the other foot forming an angle with the calcaneus. The talus points *downward* rather than forward and the navicular lies on the superior surface of the neck of the talus instead of anterior to the head.

Correction of this condition requires a series of plaster casts to change the convexity of the arch and to return the navicular to its normal place. Surgery is frequently needed to accomplish this but, with either method of treatment, the results are frequently disappointing and surgical arthrodesis is required in later life if the foot becomes painful.

Acquired Flatfoot

The acquired flatfoot is usually flexible and may appear well formed when not weight bearing or when standing on tiptoes. The foot pronates when weight bearing and assumes a flattened appearance. The longitudinal arch becomes effaced, the navicular depresses towards the floor, and the calcaneus undergoes eversion. The medial border loses its concavity and actually appears to bulge. If the flatfoot is mobile, it regains much of its longitudinal arch upon arising on tiptoes.

Children with pronated feet develop an awkward gait. They walk "toeing out" and lack "spring" in their gait. Later they may complain of aching in their calf and leg muscles. It is this complaint or the parental concern over the awkward gait that brings them to the doctor.

Pronation may be associated with generalized ligamentous laxity in which case the child also has excessive mobility in the hips, knees, elbows, and low back. This patient is often referred to as "double-jointed" as an expression of hyperextensibility. Hypo-flexibility may also cause pronation when tightness of the tendo Achillis causes pronation of the foot to permit full weight bearing. Discovery of a tight Achilles tendon during the examination reveals the cause of the pronation.

Internal Tibial Torsion

Moderate to severe internal tibial torsion may cause the foot to evert in weight bearing to compensate the torsion and allow the foot to face straight ahead. The "toe-in" stance is partially corrected by the eversion of the forefoot but this causes the foot to pronate. Internal rotation of the tibia rarely persists after infancy. It is estimated that only 10 per cent of children reaching the age of five have residual internal tibial torsion, and less than 5 per cent continue to have rotation into adolescence. Since internal rotation of the legs, especially internal tibial torsion, is usually gone by adulthood, no treatment is necessary other than elimination and avoidance of obvious postural and positional factors in the newborn state.

Pronation can be acquired after prolonged bed rest or after prolonged immobilization of the foot and leg in a plaster cast, but it is more frequently the result of faulty sleeping habits during the first four months of life. The child sleeps prone with the legs in a frog position (Fig. 56B), the hips flexed, abducted, and externally rotated. The firm mattress and bulky diapers encourage this posture. In this position all the pressure is imposed upon the inner border of the foot causing pronation. The foot invertors are thus stretched and the evertors permitted to shorten. The mechanism of pronation is instituted.

The external rotators of the hips are normally stronger than the internal rotators and this encourages the child to sit on the floor with the hips externally rotated and the feet under him. There is a tendency, however, to sit in this position with the feet turned outward, and the floor pressure against the inner border of the feet tends to pronate them.

TREATMENT OF THE PRONATED FOOT

Positioning

Treatment of the pronated foot must be considered before the child walks and be continued when walking begins. Pre-walking treatment consists of altering the faulty sleeping posture, gaining and maintaining flexibility of internal rotation of the entire leg, and exercising the foot to acquire an inverted supinated foot with a longitudinal arch. Specific ways of doing these must be carefully outlined to the parents.

The newborn child cannot be forced to sleep on its back without danger of regurgitation of the food and its aspiration, but it may be possible to cause the child to sleep on his side by propping with pillows. Frequent observation during the night and nap time are obviously required to maintain this position. Thick and multiple diapers must be avoided to minimize the frog position. If the external rotators of the hip are tight, they should be stretched many times daily by the mother. This is done with the child lying on his back with the legs extended. The mother grasps the lower thighs, rotates both legs inwardly as far as they will go, and holds them in this position for 30 to 40 seconds. This exercise should be repeated several times daily and the mother must be instructed that *stretching is the intention.* Each exercise should attempt further internal rotation until flexibility is achieved.

Exercises

The foot must be exercised to force it into adduction and supination to form a longitudinal arch. The mother must be taught how to stretch the foot and advised to do it frequently and patiently. After each stretching treatment, the foot should be held in the newly-acquired position for 30 to

45 seconds which insures that the foot will remain flexible. This period is arbitrary but gives the mother a time factor as a goal. Figure 60 demonstrates the maneuver required to form the longitudinal arch. An adult foot has been used in the illustration for clarity. In treating the child's foot the hand positions may need to be altered to fit the smaller foot, but the principles remain the same.

The child with pronated feet frequently walks awkwardly, toeing out and with no "spring" in his gait. Later in life this child frequently develops aching in the legs and curtails his activities which causes greater pronation as a result of disuse and deconditioning.

Children who exhibit tibial torsion may stand with their feet pronated although they walk with a toe-in gait. The stance with the foot facing straight ahead is done by everting and pronating the foot. Their toe-in gait permits them to bear weight on the lateral border of their foot and causes the foot to supinate and form a longitudinal arch. Toe-in gait in this condition *should be encouraged* and not discouraged or corrected. This compensatory gait occurs naturally and strengthens the foot, improves the arch, and ultimately leads to a good painless gait. The tendency to place lateral wedges on the sole and heel of the shoes to correct the toeing in should be discouraged as they merely enhance pronation of the foot.

.Treatment of the pronated foot must provide support for the longitudinal arch and must attempt to cause supination. The obese phlegmatic child should be made to lose weight and be encouraged to exercise. Proper

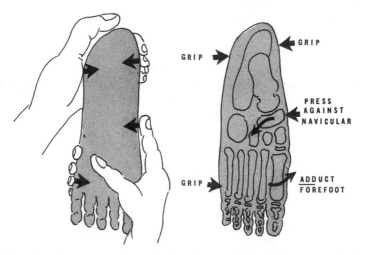

FIGURE 60. Forming an arch in a flatfoot by stretching. Illustration depicts the technique of stretching the right foot. The heel is gripped by the *left* hand holding the calcaneus in a neutral position. The index finger of the *right* hand presses against the navicular bone while the fingers of the *right* hand adduct the forefoot around the fulcrum of the index finger pressing the navicular area. For the left foot the procedure is reversed. In the illustration the right foot is viewed from above.

walking is the best exercise for these patients, and they must not be allowed to indulge their tendency to avoid walking.

Shoe Corrections

For the newborn no shoes are indicated, and when there is an abnormality present no shoe is "corrective." Correction consists of exercise, plaster casts, or even braces. A shoe can only maintain a correction once flexibility has been gained and assist in improving the gait.

The normal foot should be fitted with a blucher type shoe having a broad toe, lacing across a tongue, and preferably a low quarter (Fig. 29). A high-top shoe offers no support and does not "strengthen" the foot or the ankle. If correction is sought, the shoe last must be formed in the manner and direction desired. In the pronated foot, the sole of the shoe, the *last,* should turn in, and the counter should grip the heel in a snug fit. Any correction incorporated into the shoe will be ineffectual if the heel is free to move about the counter (Fig. 61). Pronation may also be partially corrected by elevating the inner side of the heel $\frac{1}{16}$ to $\frac{3}{16}$ in. The exact elevation will depend upon the severity of the heel valgus (Fig. 62). A Thomas heel is frequently prescribed to carry the medial counter forward and give a more anterior pivot point to help supinate the foot during walking.

The shank of the shoe should not be too firm and inflexible. A completely inflexible shank prevents normal use of the intrinsic muscles of the

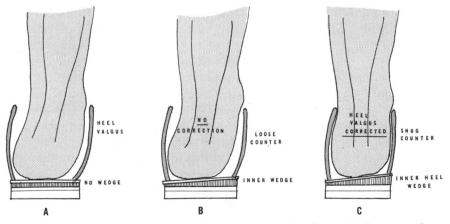

FIGURE 61. Necessity of snug heel in correcting heel valgus. A shows a valgus heel within a regular shoe. B shows that an inner wedge in the heel of a loose-fitting shoe does *not* correct the valgus. To be effective an inner wedge has to be placed on a shoe counter that "hugs" the heel, C.

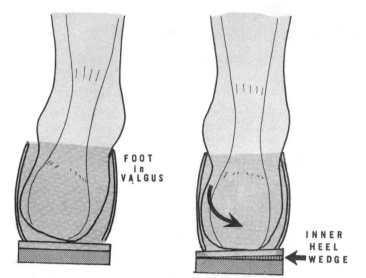

FOOT
in
VALGUS

INNER
HEEL
WEDGE

FIGURE 62. Inner heel wedge in treatment of heel valgus. The inner wedge should taper from no elevation at the outer border to 1/16 to 3/16 in. on the inner border. The exact elevation is determined by the height needed to place the calcaneus in a near-vertical position.

foot and defeats the purpose of any correction. A high-top shoe has merely the advantage of being difficult for the child to remove.

Supports

If pronation is severe and the longitudinal arch totally depressed but the foot is flexible, an arch support may be considered. The supports are molded over a plaster mold of the foot to conform to the exact contour desired for the specific foot. Made of felt or sponge rubber covered with leather, the supports tend to deform or compress under the weight of the patient and must be replaced frequently. A rigid arch may be made of metal or plastic, but it frequently causes pressure discomfort. The longitudinal arch support must elevate the arch with its apex under the navicular. The support must extend forward to end behind the first three metatarsal heads, must taper laterally to present no elevation under the lateral border of the foot, and must extend backward to end just anterior to the calcaneal weight-bearing edge. It must form the contour of a symmetrical arch and be comfortable.

A plastic arch support based upon the principle that the weight-bearing foot *supinates* when the leg rotates externally (Fig. 54) and forms a longitudinal arch has been designed by the Biomechanics Laboratory of the University of California. A mold of the foot is made from a plastic plaster applied skintight over a thin rubber covering. The foot is then placed on a rotating platform and the leg, with the foot weight bearing, is externally rotated. The mold hardens in this supinated position. Using a positive cast made from the mold, the arch support is made of a fiber glass material. The support fits the heel snugly thus maintaining the acquired vertical position of the calcaneus, and the forefoot is held in supination by the medial and lateral phalanges (Fig. 63). This technique is not yet known by many orthotists and may be difficult to procure, but it is based on sound physiological principles and should ultimately receive wide acceptance.

Gait Training

Exercise is the most beneficial form of treatment of the pronated foot. Corrective shoes and arch supports are essentially "crutches" to be considered as a means to an end and not ends in themselves. The exercises must be modified according to the age of the child and his ability to cooperate. The heel cord must be sufficiently extensible to permit more than 90 degrees of dorsiflexion (Fig. 41). The gastroc-soleus group must be strong and can be strengthened by exercises such as rising on the toes or walking on tiptoes.

The intrinsic muscles of the foot can be strengthened by toe-flexor exercises such as picking up marbles, wrinkling a towel lying on the floor, or standing on the outer border of both feet and actively flexing the toes while in this position.

FIGURE 63. The uc-bl shoe insert. The laminated fiber glass insert shell is molded over a plaster mold of the foot. It fits snugly into the shoe. The heel is held in a neutral position and the forefoot held in an adducted supinated position.

69

Teaching a child to walk with a heel-toe gait and the feet turned out about 10 degrees may, by constant repetition, result in his adopting this method as the subconscious manner of walking. In the very severe case where toeing in (or out) cannot be voluntarily controlled or exists in a child too young to cooperate, "twisters" (Fig. 64) may be used.

Toe-in gait, commonly called "pigeon-toed," may result from excessive anteversion of the femoral neck (Fig. 36), congenital hip dislocation, knock-knee, marked internal tibial torsion, or metatarsus varus. The exact patho-mechanics of the gait must be discovered and, if possible, be corrected.

METATARSUS VARUS

Metatarsus varus is a common condition in newborns (Fig. 65). This condition is also termed metatarsus adductus and some would differentiate the two terms, but they are sufficiently similar to use the names interchangeably.

FIGURE 64. Orthotic "twisters" to control internal or external rotation. The "twisters" are coiled springs within a cable housing that resists torque. By its attachment at the pelvic band and to the shoe the foot can be made to turn *in* or *out* by adjustment. It permits ambulation and controls the rotation both in stance and swing phase of walking.

ADDUCTED FOREFOOT

VALGUS HEEL

FIGURE 65. Metatarsus varus. The foot in metatarsus varus has an adducted forefoot, a convex lateral foot border, and the heel is in valgus. No equinus is present.

Diagnosis

Metatarsus varus is not a severe deformity but the child may walk in an awkward manner, he toes in and frequently "trips" over his own feet. He wears out his shoes early and distorts them. This condition may be adequately corrected but recurrences are frequent, and correction without adequate and prolonged follow-up leads to failure.

The following components of metatarsus varus (Fig. 66) must be recognized to establish proper diagnosis and to ensure adequate treatment: (1) the anterior segment of the foot is in *adduction,* (2) the lateral border of the foot is convex with the apex of the convexity appearing at the base of the fifth metatarsal, (3) the heel is in *valgus,* (4) internal tibial torsion is frequently present, (5) there is a sharp angulation of the medial border of the foot at the tarsometatarsal joint, (6) the first metatarsal is more angulated than the other four but all are angulated, (7) the talus is medially

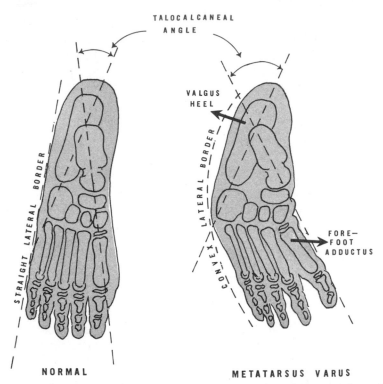

FIGURE 66. Components of metatarsus varus compared to the normal foot. Metatarsus varus has an adducted forefoot and a valgus heel. The lateral margin of the foot is convex with the apex at the base of the fifth metatarsal. The talus is medially and anteriorly displaced in relationship to the calcaneus thus increasing the talo calcaneal angle.

and anteriorly displaced in its relation to the calcaneus, and (8) there is no equinus and no limitation of dorsiflexion as is seen in talipes equinovarus or "clubfoot."

Treatment

Treatment should be instituted early. In many cases the condition corrects itself in time, but the large percentage of cases in which it persists and causes cosmetic and slight functional impairment justifies early vigorous treatment. Exercises administered by the parents are usually ineffectual. A Denis Browne splint has the danger of everting the feet thus accentuating the heel valgus without correcting the forefoot. Reversing the shoes by putting the right on the left foot and vice versa may hold the mild flexible metatarsus varus in a corrected position but does not correct the moderate or severe adductus. A series of plaster casts that simultaneously correct the forefoot and the hindfoot have been found effective. The heel is forced medially, the calcaneus moves under the talus, and the heel is placed into the varus position. This maneuver requires pressure upon the cuboid while moving the calcaneus and the forefoot is simultaneously forced into abduction (Fig. 67). Pronation of the forefoot must be avoided. Before the cast is permitted to dry fully the transverse metatarsal arch can be molded into slight dorsal convexity (Fig. 12). Each cast should be left on for two weeks before it is replaced by a cast that attempts further correction. Casting is continued until the foot is slightly *overcorrected*.

The cast is applied with the foot in slight equinus and in slight inversion to the long axis of the leg. The toes should be left exposed. The position of the heel is better controlled if the cast extends above the knee which also permits external rotation of the leg to correct any associated internal tibial torsion.

Metatarsus varus must not be confused with talipes equinovarus ("club-foot"). In metatarsus varus the heel is in the valgus position whereas in

FIGURE 67. Technique of manipulating metatarsus varus. Illustration shows the method of correcting metatarsus varus during plaster casting. Pressure, C, against the cuboid and anterior portion of the calcaneus medially forces the calcaneus under the talus and thus corrects the valgus. H is traction on the posterior aspect of the calcaneus to aid C in moving the calcaneus into a neutral or varus position. F is simultaneous pressure by the other hand to correct the adducted metatarsals. All pressures are applied simultaneously.

talipes equinovarus it is in varus. The clubfoot is in equinus and resists dorsiflexion due to contracted posterior leg muscles. The metatarsus varus has free dorsiflexion and the foot can be dorsiflexed sufficiently to bring the dorsum of the foot in contact with the tibia. In the metatarsus varus foot the calcaneus can usually be moved easily into the varus position whereas in clubfoot the heel is "fixed" in the varus position.

METATARSUS PRIMUS VARUS

Diagnosis

Metatarsus primus varus is a condition that mimics metatarsus varus but only the first metatarsal is in adduction and all the other metatarsals are in proper alignment. The first metatarsal is angulated medially upon the medial cuneiform or may be aligned to a deformed cuneiform (Fig. 68). The lateral border of the foot does not show the convexity noted in metatarsus varus. Treatment is usually unnecessary.

TALIPES EQUINOVARUS (CONGENITAL CLUBFOOT)

Talipes equinovarus, commonly termed "clubfoot," is considered the most significant congenital fixed deformity of the foot. Found more commonly in boys than in girls, it is considered a defect in prenatal development and may occur in one or both feet.

Diagnosis

The condition is characterized by the following components: (1) inversion (*twisting inward*) and adduction (*inward deviation*) of the forefoot (Fig. 69), (2) varus of the calcaneus (*inversion of the heel*), (3) equinus (*plantar flexion*), (4) contraction of the tissues on the medial side of the foot, (5) underdeveloped evertor muscles on the lateral side of the leg, (6) underdeveloped and contracted calf muscles, and (7) resistance to passive correction.

A plantar flexed inverted foot in the newborn that cannot be brought into a dorsiflexed or everted position suggests talipes equinovarus. This is contrary to the normal child's foot that may be plantar flexed and inverted but is completely flexible. If differs from the metatarsus varus foot in which the heel is in valgus and mobile. In clubfoot the toes also are flexed and resist extension and there is usually an associated internal tibial torsion. The child stands bearing his weight on the base of the fifth metatarsal bone.

MET ATARSUS
VARUS
PRIMUS

ANGLED
MEDIAL
CUNEIFORM

NORMAL
TALOCALCANEAL
ANGLE

FIGURE 68. Metatarsus primus varus. Primus varus grossly resembles metatarsus varus but in primus only the first metatarsal is in adduction. The remaining metatarsals are in proper alignment. The first metatarsal may adduct because of a deformed medial cuneiform or may be angled medially upon a normal cuneiform. The talocalcaneal angle reveals no deviation of the talar relationship upon the calcaneus.

Treatment

Treatment must be instituted immediately after birth by corrective plaster casting. Time is of the essence and procrastination by instituting ineffectual massage, corrective shoes, and passive exercises only delays proper treatment and decreases the probability of correction.

Prognosis relative to the degree of improvement is guarded as the tissues creating the deformity are atrophic, fibrosed, and contracted. There is also an irreversible muscular imbalance. Treatment aims to prevent bony and articular deformity and to minimize fibrous contracture. Recurrence is possible even after adequate correction in early childhood thus a long term program of observation and treatment must be instituted. The initial treatment is to correct, then to overcorrect, and maintain the corrected position

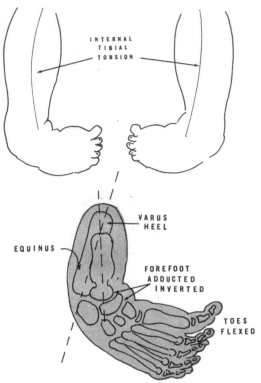

FIGURE 69. Talipes equinovarus: "clubfoot." Talipes equinovarus or clubfoot has an inflexible adducted forefoot and a varus heel. The toes are usually flexed. The medial tissues of the foot and ankle are contracted, the Achilles tendon is shortened, and there is usually some internal tibial torsion. These deformities resist passive stretching.

of the foot until bone structure is fully developed. Recurrence then is less likely to occur.

Casts applied to the newborn are changed at each stage of correction. If the child is over two months of age, the initial casts can safely be wedged. The cast should be applied to the foot covered with a thin layer of Webril or felt so that the contours can be molded yet the bony prominences protected. Correction is made by firm manual pressure *correcting the adductus* and *inversion first* and making *no attempt to alter the equinus.* The cast should be molded carefully and should not be modified once the plaster has begun to set. Alteration after partial drying may cause wrinkling of the cast forming pressure points against vulnerable areas of the foot. A faulty or unsatisfactory cast is best removed and reapplied.

Attempting correction of equinus concurrently with correction of the adductus and inversion may result in the formation of a "rocker bottom." 'Rocker bottom" implies reversal of the longitudinal arch with a convex rather than concave plantar surface. The equinus calf contracture resists elongation, and efforts to correct the equinus initially may cause dorsiflexion of the forefoot upon the hind foot and reverses of the longitudinal arch.

Casts are applied and changed once or twice a week, first correcting the adducted forefoot and ultimately achieving overcorrection. The calcaneus is brought under the talus and the heel placed in the valgus position. The cast is extended to include the flexed knee which controls the position sought for the heel.

The contracted Achilles becomes more resistant to elongation by this delay, but the forefoot must be corrected to prevent recurrence and to minimize the formation of a rocker bottom. Once the adductus and inversion are overcorrected the equinus is gradually corrected by progressive dorsiflexion of the ankle.

Internal tibial torsion may be corrected by externally rotating the leg since the plaster cast extends to include the flexed knee. A Denis Browne type of splint may be incorporated into the plaster casts of the feet to gain external rotation and abduction, but the use of a Denis Browne splint without plaster casting the feet will not correct the major deformities of the heel and forefoot.

The foot once corrected can be maintained in this acquired position by bivalved plaster casts or by corrective shoes externally rotated on a Denis Browne bar (Fig. 70). Surgical correction is indicated if correction has not been achieved within four months by casting. There currently is a

DENIS BROWNE SPLINT

FIGURE 70. The Denis Browne splint. The spreader bar which may be metal, plastic, or wood is firmly attached to a pair of shoes. The shoe attachment may be fixed or adjustable so that the shoes can be turned in or out, everted or inverted, as the need dictates. The width of the spreader bar depends on the desired abduction of the legs and hips.

tendency to operate earlier to re-establish the normal relationship of the tarsal bones and to remove the deforming forces of muscles and soft tissues. Instances of recurrence are claimed to be less with early surgical intervention, but as yet conclusive evidence is lacking.

Operative procedures involve the following: (1) soft tissue release of medial border tissues and lengthening of the tendo Achillis, (2) tendon transplants to change evertors to invertors and dorsiflexors. The anterior tibial tendon, which is basically an invertor-dorsiflexor, is transferred laterally to the base of the third metatarsal to become an evertor. The posterior tibial, a powerful plantar flexor-invertor, is released or is transferred laterally, (3) osteotomy or arthrodesis in which the bones and their joints are remolded and fused in the newly acquired position. In later life triple arthrodesis may be necessary to reform the foot. Detailed discussion of operative techniques is not included in this text. The reader is referred to current literature where they are well documented.

When the child begins to walk, exercises are begun to maintain the elongated position of the gastroc-soleus group and the evertors. Exercises to strengthen underdeveloped gastrocnemius and peronei muscles should be daily ritual. Shoes for clubfoot and lateral sole and heel wedges will improve the gait and maintain the corrected forefoot and heel position.

TARSAL COALITION

Rigid flatfoot is frequently caused by an anomalous fusion of two or more tarsal bones. This coalition prevents movement between the two tarsal bones involved causing a static foot deformity. The fusion may be osseous, cartilaginous, or fibrous. The most common coalitions exist between the talus and calcaneus and between the calcaneus and the navicular (Fig. 71).

Diagnosis

Tarsal coalition may be asymptomatic. It probably exists from birth but rarely gives symptoms until late adolescence or early adulthood when trauma such as prolonged standing, prolonged marching, or jumping may induce symptoms. The pain undoubtedly results from the stress sustained by the remaining functioning joints due to the unyielding coalition.

X-rays of the osseous bridge are requested when the clinical picture suggests coalition as a possible diagnosis. Cartilaginous or fibrous coalitions are not seen on the X-rays but are assumed from clinical evaluation of a rigid painful foot that does not respond to conservative treatment.

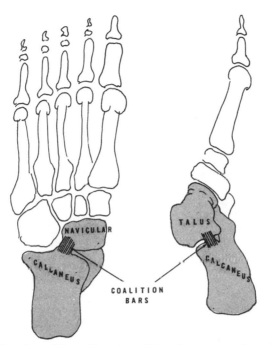

FIGURE 71. Tarsal coalition. Tarsal coalition is an anomalous fusion of two or more tarsal bones by a bony, cartilaginous, or fibrous bar. The commonest types are talocalcaneal and calcanconavicular. Their presence may form a rigid flatfoot or a peroneal "spastic" flatfoot. When the bar is bone it can be visualized on X-ray otherwise its presence is diagnosed clinically.

Treatment

If trauma has produced mild discomfort, treatment is symptomatic and includes rest with heat applications. Immobilization of the foot and ankle in a walking plaster cast may be indicated to give complete rest and yet permit ambulation. If the coalition is considered to be the cause of the disability and persistent pain, resection of the bar or fusion stabilization of the subtalar joints may be necessary.

CONGENITAL VERTICAL TALUS

This uncommon condition should be suspected when the foot of the newborn is fixed in equinus and abduction. As the foot is dorsiflexed the head of the talus forms a prominence at the expected longitudinal arch concavity similar to a rocker bottom foot and resembles a clubfoot improperly casted. X-rays reveal the vertical talus.

Treatment

Treatment by manipulation and plaster casting is indicated but unfortunately is usually disappointing. The improvement is often merely in the appearance but not in the function of the foot. Surgical correction offers the most benefit.

BIBLIOGRAPHY

Adams, J. C.: Outline of Orthopaedics, ed. 5. The Williams & Wilkins Co., Baltimore, 1964.

Cailliet, R.: Bracing for Spasticity. In Orthotics Etcetera. Physical Medicine Library, Vol. 9, edited by S. Licht. Elizabeth Licht Publisher, New Haven, 1966, p. 365.

Du Vries, H. L.: Surgery of the Foot, ed. 2. The C. V. Mosby Co., St. Louis, 1965.

Gartland, J. J.: Fundamentals of Orthopaedics. W. B. Saunders Co., Philadelphia, 1965.

Hark, F. W.: Rocker-Foot Due to Congenital Subluxation of the Talus. J. Bone Joint Surg. 32A:344, 1950.

Henderson, W. H., and Campbell, J. W.: The UC-BL Shoe Insert; Casting and Fabrication. Biomechanics Laboratory of the University of California, July 1964.

Hutter, C. G., and Scott, W.: Tibial Torsion. J. Bone Joint Surg. 31-A:511, 1949.

Kite, J. H.: Congenital Metatarsus Varus. Report of 300 Cases. J. Bone Joint Surg. 32-A: 500, 1950.

Kite, J. H.: Shoes for Children. Orthotics Etcetera. Physical Medicine Library, Vol. 9, edited by S. Licht. Elizabeth Licht, Publisher, New Haven, 1966, p. 453.

Leibolt, F. L.: Shoes for Children, Symposium in Pediatric Orthopedics, Pediatric Clinics of North America, W. B. Saunders Co., Philadelphia, 1955.

Lewin, P.: The Foot and Ankle, ed. 4. Lea & Febiger, Philadelphia, 1959.

MacConaill, M. A.: The Postural Mechanism of the Human Foot. Proc. Roy. Irish Acad. 1B:265, May 1945.

McCauley, J., Jr., Luskin, R., and Bromley, J.: Recurrence in Congenital Metatarsus Varus. J. Bone Joint Surg. 46-A:525, 1964.

Norton, P. L.: Pediatric Orthopedics. Symposium in Pediatric Orthopedics, Pediatric Clinics of North America, W. B. Saunders Co., Philadelphia, 1955.

Ponseti, I. V., and Becker, J. R.: Congenital Metatarsus Adductus. The Results of Treatment. J. Bone Joint Surg. 48-A:702, 1966.

Vaughn, W. H., and Segal, G.: Tarsal Coalition with Special Reference to Roentgenographic Interpretation. Radiology. 60:855, 1953.

Webster, F. S., and Roberts, W. M.: Tarsal Anomalies and Peroneal Spastic Flatfoot, J.A.M.A. 146:1099, 1951.

CHAPTER 5

Painful Disorders of the Adult Foot

NORMAL FOOT

The *normal foot* conforms to the following criteria: (1) pain free, (2) normal muscle balance, (3) absence of contracture, (4) three-point weight bearing, (5) a central heel, and (6) straight and mobile toes.

The majority of painful conditions of the foot originate in the soft tissues: the muscles, ligaments, tendons, nerves, and blood vessels. Articular and skeletal causes may be present from congenital abnormalities, infections, neoplasms, or trauma, but even in these cases the early symptoms come from soft-tissue changes.

In most cases of foot and ankle pain, the symptoms can be explained by local lesions. Usually the area of pain pointed out by the patient specifies its exact anatomical site. The history gives the mechanism producing pain. Only rarely is foot pain referred from a proximal site, but the examiner must be aware that a local disturbance, such as a flatfoot, may be an incidental finding in cases where the pain is referred.

FOOT STRAIN

Foot strain may be acute, subacute, or chronic. It may occur in the normal foot from normal walking or standing if the patient has been unaccustomed to a great deal of activity. Since foot strain has a mechanical effect on the soft tissues, if it is allowed to persist, deformity may result. A foot considered mechanically abnormal may be strained by essentially normal activity. Stress on a pre-existing deformity will cause earlier and more intense pain and the foot will resist correction and palliation. The general rule that applies to all musculo-skeletal dysfunctions applies here; that is, pain and dysfunction can occur from (1) abnormal stress on a normal structure, (2) normal stress on an abnormal structure, or (3) normal stress on a normal structure when the structure is not prepared for the stress.

The static foot is supported by ligamentous tissues. There is no muscular activity in the foot or leg muscles during standing even when large weights are superimposed upon the body. The muscular activity during locomotion prevents excessive strain upon the supportive ligaments and joint tissues. Therefore, pain in the static foot must result from faulty mechanics or an overwhelming stress upon the ligaments. In the moving foot, pain results when muscular incompetence due to disuse, imbalance, or abuse places an excessive burden upon the ligaments. In either case, the stress upon the soft tissues causes inflammation, elongation, and ultimately degeneration of the ligaments.

Acute Foot Strain

Acute painful ligamentous strain is usually self-limited, subsides with rest, and rarely presents a therapeutic problem. The acute situation is exemplified in the person paying an unaccustomed visit to a museum, the weekend athlete, or the doctor visiting the many booths at an annual convention. Rest followed by a gradual return to normal activities leads to recovery.

Chronic Foot Strain

If excessive stress is repeated or if normal stress is imposed upon a mechanical abnormality, the symptoms may become chronic. Symptoms may vary from those of ligamentous strain to those caused by joint malalignment resulting from the stress. Ultimately degenerative arthritic changes may be the source of pain.

The "breakdown" process follows a sequence. Ligaments exposed to chronic strain elongate and undergo inflammatory changes which result in pain. If the condition persists, the ligaments elongate and degenerate, lose their supporting function, and permit excessive motion of the joints. This excessive "play" and misalignment of the joints will inflame the joint capsules and surfaces, and articular inflammation becomes the source of pain. If irritation to the joints continues, structural damage to the articular surfaces results, and degenerative arthritis is present. Nature responds to these irritations by attempting reconstruction or forming a bulwark against the irritation with an overgrowth of bone that results in a deformed joint called an "arthrosis." If early changes are recognized, this cycle is reversible, but if it is allowed to proceed too far, the joint may be beyond repair.

The initial symptom of acute stress from activity such as prolonged walking is muscular fatigue usually described as an "aching" in the sole of the foot, in the calf muscles, or occasionally in the anterior leg. Deep tenderness of the plantar tissues of the foot or the leg muscles is found. The foot, now symptomatic, may be normal but is more likely to be a pronated foot which flattens its longitudinal arch upon weight bearing. Muscular fatigue from activity permits stress to be imposed upon the ligaments resulting in ligamentous pain (Fig. 72).

Mechanism and Sequence

The mechanism and sequence by which strain is imposed upon the areas of the foot are illustrated in (Fig. 73 and 74). The foot and ankle must be considered as a complex structure with each of its component parts dependent upon the others. Body weight is borne upon the talus through its articulation with the tibia. In turn, the talus is supported by the calcaneus and is held in an oblique manner. The oblique seating of the

FIGURE 72. Tender areas in foot strain. "Trigger areas" noted in the foot undergoing strain. The initial tenderness is usually noted on the medial border of the plantar fascia and later near the heel. The deltoid ligament is not shown but is a point of tenderness near the posterior tibial tendon which becomes strained. The second metatarsal head is the most prevalent site of metatarsalgia.

FIGURE 73. Mechanism and sequence of foot strain. The upper figures depict the normal foot with proper bone and joint alignment, adequate longitudinal arch, and a central heel, 1. The weight-bearing stress imparted through the tibia upon the talus, 2, which slides forward and medially, 5, upon the supporting calcaneus. The calcaneus, 3, is depressed anteriorly elongating the entire foot, thus placing strain upon the plantar ligaments, 4. The calcaneus everts under the downward pressure of the talus and goes into valgus, 6.

talus upon the calcaneus gives the talus a tendency to *glide forward* and *medially upon the calcaneus*. The resultant force of this movement forces the calcaneus into eversion and depresses its anterior portion. This pronation depresses the longitudinal arch and stretches the plantar ligament and fascia.

The valgus position of the heel places a torque stress upon the forefoot which responds by becoming everted. The foot now bears the weight on its inner border which forces the foot into more pronation thus placing strain on the medial ankle ligaments and upon the tendon of the posterior tibial muscle. Due to the valgus heel position the Achilles tendon deviates laterally and shortens. The shortened tendon places more strain upon the anterior segments of the foot.

Pronation

This sequence of effects of foot strain may be imposed upon a normal foot but is more apt to occur in the already pronated or deconditioned foot.

FIGURE 74. Mechanism of foot strain: superior view. The heel is forced into valgus from the downward pressure of the superincumbant talus, 2. This causes the forefoot to abduct (evert) and spread out, 7. The normal transverse arch flattens and depresses the central metatarsal heads, 8.

As the protective muscular action is overwhelmed, the stress is imparted upon the ligaments, then the joint capsules, and ultimately the joints. Joints so strained separate slightly, and the foot undergoes a functional deformity. Persistence of the stress ultimately converts the functional deformity into a structural one. Recovery from an acute strain is brief if the tissues are healthy and mobile. If the strain is chronic or the tissues are defective, deformity becomes chronic and subsequent stresses although minor can elicit major symptoms.

During the early phase of strain upon the foot, the muscles acting across the foot attempt to allay the strain upon the ligaments. They may react to this stress with pain. The posterior tibial, as the prime invertor of the foot, opposes the eversion of the foot, and its tendon may become inflamed and tender. On examination, tenderness of the posterior tibial tendon can be elicited by palpation along its course under and behind the medial malleolus (Fig. 72). The long flexor of the big toe, which has a function similar to the posterior tibial and also presses the toe to the ground, also becomes strained and painfully inflamed.

As the foot and forefoot go more into pronation, the lateral evertors must shorten to take up the slack. The peronei muscles and toe extensors, the evertors, go into "spasm" as they undergo adaptive shortening, and they too become painful and tender.

The interosseous talocalcaneal ligament which binds the talus to the calcaneus (Fig. 8) is normally taut when the foot is supinated and slack when the foot is pronated. As the strained foot pronates, the tarsal canal deforms and the talocalcaneal joint becomes abnormally mobile. Although slack, the interosseous ligament undergoes strain with ultimate inflammation. This tender ligament can be palpated at the lateral orifice of the sinus canal just anterior to the lateral malleolus (Fig. 40). Tenderness of this ligament occurs late in the sequence as the foot undergoes pronation deformity.

Early ligamentous symptoms are felt on the plantar surface of the foot (Fig. 72) with the areas of tenderness palpable in the plantar fascia, the medial ligaments of the ankle at their attachment to the sustentaculum talus (Fig. 6 and 39), and the posterior tibial tendon passing under the medial malleolus.

Diagnosis

The early signs and symptoms in the soft tissues which relate to structural surface anatomy (Fig. 38, 39, and 40) are pointed to by the patient and ascertained by the examiner. Functional anatomy gives a mechanical explanation by which abnormal function results in pain and disability. It is evident that pronation is a major cause of pain, and that deconditioning as well as excessive stress initiates a process of decompensation. This emphasizes the need for a long-range program of treatment for children with markedly pronated feet to allay ultimate pain and disability in adulthood.

The toe flexors, as well as the supinators of the foot, play a vital role in the maintenance of the longitudinal and transverse arches. Balance between the toe flexors and extensors must exist for proper foot function. Normally the extensor digitorum longus and the lumbricals extend the distal interphalangeal joints (Fig. 75) and the toe flexors press the straightened toes against the floor. This action elevates the transverse arch. If the intrinsics are weak, the phalanges are permitted to flex, and the action of the toe flexors causes a "claw" position of the toes. The metatarsal heads become more prominent and weight bearing. With weakness of the toe flexors the downward pressure upon the floor is also weakened.

The excessive joint "play" resulting from ligamentous laxity causes pain due to articular strain. The calcaneocuboid and the talonavicular joints (Fig. 76) sustain this stress primarily by virtue of the foot pronating and the forefoot everting.

Pain originating from articular strain does not subside with rest as does pain from ligamentous, tendinous, or muscular origin. No "trigger" areas

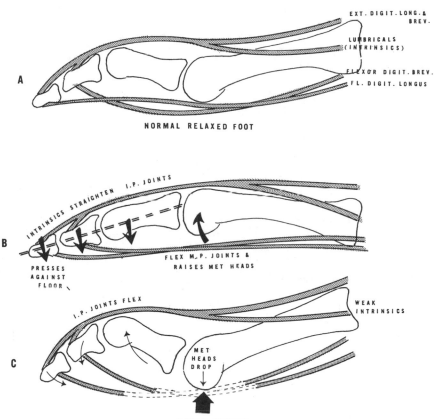

FIGURE 75. Muscular mechanism forming transverse arch. The transverse arch is only a potential arch, not an anatomical arch. The metatarsal heads are raised by the toes being kept straight and the metatarso-phalangeal joints being flexed, B, by the long and short flexors. Weakness of the intrinsics permits the toes to bend at the interphalangeal joints and the flexors then increase the flexion at the interphalangeal joints. The metatarsal heads thus bear the full-body weight.

are palpable, and the patient points to a region overlying the joint involved. Pain can be reproduced by forcefully everting the forefoot while immobilizing the heel.

Talonavicular arthrosis resulting from chronic foot strain causes tenderness over the dorsum of the foot at the talonavicular joint, and because the navicular is depressed in the pronated foot, there is also tenderness on the plantar surface of the foot at the calcaneonavicular ligament.

Treatment

Treatment of foot strain is essentially the treatment of the adult flatfoot. In acute strain, rest is desirable and walking must be curtailed or completely

ABDUCTION
OF
FOREFOOT

CALCANEO-
CUBOID
ARTHROSIS

NAVICULAR
DEPRESSED

TALONAVICULAR
ARTHROSIS

FIGURE 76. The chronically strained foot. The abducted forefoot of the chronically strained foot causes articular changes due to pressure of the abducted cuboid upon the calcaneus. The talus drops and causes pressure upon the superior portion of the navicular. Mechanical pressures at joints cause arthrosis.

eliminated. Application of heat or cold may be used depending upon which affords the greater relief. Early use of cold, and later the use of heat is generally preferred. The use of alternating hot and cold baths is soothing. Stimulation of the plantar muscles with faradic current allegedly affords comfort by decreasing the soft-tissue inflammation. When the symptoms are sufficiently severe or fail to respond to brief rest, immobilization of the foot in a plaster cast may be indicated. A cast removes all stress from the intrinsic muscles of the foot and gives total rest while still permitting ambulation.

After the acute symptoms have subsided, rehabilitation of the foot must be undertaken. Often the patient's history indicates that pain began after a change in occupation, a change in activities involving excessive standing or walking, a period of excessive weight gain, or a period of immobilization causing disuse wasting of the muscles. It is not unusual to find that symptoms began with the wearing of a different type of shoe. These factors are very often the cause of foot pain and once discovered must be altered or remedied.

Exercises similar to those given the child with pronated feet (Chapter

4) are extremely valuable for patients up to the age of fifty and can be of value even at a later stage in life. These exercises preferably are done barefooted. While seated, the patient turns the foot down, in, up, and out drawing a wide circle. This must be done forcefully with every effort to get the fullest possible range of motion. Simultaneously the toes should be alternately flexed and extended. This type of exercise elongates the tissues and strengthens the muscles of the leg and foot. Circulation is also enhanced.

Similar exercises can be performed standing. The patient stands with his feet apart and slight toeing in. Rolling to the outer border of his feet, the patient simultaneously curls the toes forcefully. Rising on the toes strengthens the calf group and the toe flexors and the patient should be encouraged to practice walking on his toes with a slight pigeon-toed gait. If the heel cord is tight, it can be stretched by the exercise shown in Figure 41 in which the patient leans forward against a wall keeping one leg behind and the forward leg not weight bearing. The posterior foot is kept facing straight ahead with the heel to the ground. As the patient leans towards the wall the Achilles tendon is stretched. The toe flexors can be exercised by wrinkling a towel lying on the floor or picking up marbles with the toes.

All the exercises prescribed are of value when done daily and systematically for long periods. The patient should do these exercises while wearing his shoes during his work day. He must be advised to walk with a slight toe-in gait and with a slight spring during push-off. Most *important of all, he must walk* increasing distances daily.

Corrective shoes in the adult seek to decrease the strain causing pronation. An adult foot in which the abnormal articular structure is fixed cannot be modified as can a child's or adult's whose foot is flexible. The shoe is modified by elevating the inner border using a Thomas heel with an inner wedge of ⅛ to ³⁄₁₆ in. An inner wedge may also be incorporated into the sole to raise the entire inner border of the shoe.

Tape with ¼-in. adhesive-backed sponge rubber can be applied to elevate the portion of the foot desired. Several layers of moleskin or felt of varying thicknesses cut into the desired pattern and taped properly to the foot is also effective (Fig. 77).

Arch supports may help rehabilitate the flexible flatfoot. They must be molded to conform to the shape of the foot that is partially weight bearing yet properly formed; they are never molded to the shape of the non-weight-bearing foot. They must be sufficiently firm to support the body weight without completely deforming. The shoe must be large enough to accommodate both the arch supports and the foot.

Shoes must be fitted properly. As foot tone is best in the morning and the foot "spreads" and slightly deforms as the day progresses, shoes should be fitted late in the day. The shoe should be broad across the forefoot, have a firm-fitting counter and have a last that conforms to the weight-

FIGURE 77.   Shoe modifications to correct strain factors.

bearing print of the foot. It should be long enough to project 1 in. ahead
of the big toe. Women's shoes should have broad low heels, rounded toes,
and a vamp that will not constrict the metatarsal heads. It is a sad commen-
tary that women's shoes are designed exclusively for style and custom with
no concern for comfort and health.

90

METATARSALGIA

Metatarsalgia is pain and tenderness of the plantar heads of the metatarsal bones which occurs when the transverse arch becomes depressed and the middle metatarsal heads bear a disproportionate amount of weight. In normal weight bearing, the first metatarsal head with its sesamoids sustains two sixths of the weight (Fig. 78) and the other heads one sixth each. The fifth metatarsal head probably bears slightly more weight than the middle heads. When the transverse arch is flattened, greater weight is borne on the second, third, and fourth metatarsal heads (Fig. 79). The dorsal and plantar interosseous ligaments which support the arch are stretched and the forefoot "splays" out.

Diagnosis

At first there is merely tenderness over the metatarsal heads to substantiate the complaint of aching pain often described as "walking with a pebble in the shoe." Later, as abnormal weight bearing continues, a callus

STATIC FOOT

FIGURE 78. Weight-bearing points of the foot. There are six weight-bearing points of the metatarsal heads. Due to the two sesamoid bones the first metatarsal carries two-sixths of the weight. This balance is upset in the pronated or splay foot.

91

FIGURE 79. Splay foot. A constitutional weakness of the intermetatarsal ligament combined with weakness of the intrinsic muscles of the foot may cause the foot to spread excessively under weight bearing. Symptoms consist of pressure pain of the middle metatarsal heads with formation of bunions and calluses.

forms to protect the exposed metatarsal heads but actually aggravates the irritation by increasing the pressure.

Metatarsalgia is most common after a weight gain in middle age. The intrinsic muscles lose their tone and the patient favors a more sedentary existence. The foot pronates in the manner described as a flatfoot and the transverse arch depresses. With the foot everted, the toe extensors function more to dorsiflex the foot and further expose the heads of the metatarsals by extending the phalanges upon the metatarsals.

Treatment

Metatarsalgia due to depressed transverse arch is treated by elevating the middle portion of the arch which avoids pressure on the painful metatarsal heads. All the aspects of treating the pronated foot must be utilized including exercises to strengthen the intrinsic muscles, Achilles tendon stretching, improvement of gait, weight reduction, and the use of appliances such as the Thomas heel, the inner heel wedge, and the metatarsal pad (Fig. 77). The metatarsal pad must be placed *behind* the metatarsal heads to relieve the pressure on them. If it is placed *under* the heads, a frequent error made by the orthotist or shoe repairman, the condition will be aggravated (Fig. 80). Calluses must be pared by soaking the foot in warm water and then using a stone or emery board. But to administer all these ancillary

92

BROAD
BLUCHER
SHOE

METATARSAL
PAD

THOMAS HEEL

SNUG
COUNTER

FIGURE 80. Shoe modifications in treatment of metatarsalgia. Placement of the metatarsal pad to elevate the heads of the second and third metatarsals must be *behind* the metatarsal heads. The broad forefoot shoe and a soft upper permits spreading of the foot without cramping, and the soft upper prevents calluses from forming on the dorsum of the toes. If a Thomas heel is used, the counter must be snug to hold the heel centrally.

forms of treatment and not correct the abnormal mechanics of the foot is to invite recurrence.

SPLAY FOOT

Splay foot is essentially a broadened forefoot due to weakness of the intermetatarsal ligaments associated with weakness of the intrinsic muscles (Fig. 79). The transverse arch flattens and the middle metatarsal heads bear more than the usual amount of weight. Calluses form on the plantar surfaces of the heads. Hammer toes may form due to the excessive extension of the toes and cause pain and tenderness on the dorsum of the toe joints. Calluses may form here. The splay foot is not a specific entity but usually accompanies the pronated foot. It more aptly applies to a broad flexible forefoot and a minor degree of pronation. Treatment is the same as for the pronated foot.

SHORT FIRST TOE: MORTON'S SYNDROME

A short first metatarsal, termed Morton's syndrome (Dudley Morton) causes excessive weight to be borne by the second metatarsal head and is usually hereditary. Morton's syndrome consists of (1) an excessively short first metatarsal, which is hypermobile at its base where it articulates with the second metatarsal and the cuneiform, (2) posterior displacement of the sesamoids, and (3) thickening of the second metatarsal shaft (Fig. 81).

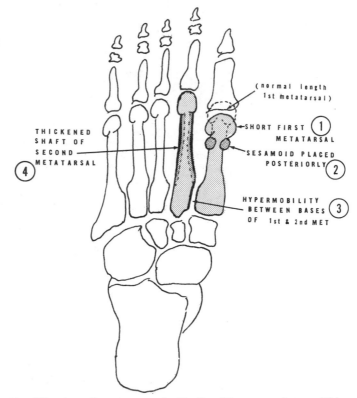

FIGURE 81. The short first metatarsal: Dudley Morton syndrome. This syndrome of metatarsalgia consists of, 1, a shorter than normal first metatarsal, 2, posterior displacement of the sesamoid bones, 3, excessive mobility of the first metatarsal at its base and, 4, thickening of the shaft of the second metatarsal due to excessive weight bearing imposed upon this bone. The pain and tenderness is usually felt at the *base* of the first two metatarsals and the *head* of the second.

Diagnosis

The additional weight borne by the second metatarsal causes excessive mobility at its base and strain of the ligaments, capsules, and muscles where the metatarsal articulates with the cuneiform and the second metatarsal. Calluses form under the second and third metatarsals because the transverse arch is also depressed.

Treatment

Treatment consists of building a "platform" under the first metatarsal bone to assume the weight and relieve the second metatarsal. The other forms of treating pronated foot are also indicated for Morton's syndrome.

Morton's syndrome (Dudley Morton) should not be confused with Morton's metatarsalgia (Thomas G. Morton). Morton's metatarsalgia is basically a neuralgia due to an interdigital neuroma. This is a fibrous thickening of the digital nerve usually between the third and fourth metatarsals and is fully discussed in Chapter 9 (Fig. 103).

MARCH FRACTURE

Diagnosis

March fracture is a stress fracture of a metatarsal bone. Pain, often noted after a long march, is the presenting symptom. A history of violent injury is rare, making the cause difficult to pinpoint. The pathology is a hairline fracture of the shaft of the second or third metatarsal with no displacement of the fragments. Initially the fracture may not be revealed by routine X-rays, but later callous formation around the fracture is radiologically apparent (Fig. 82) and confirms the diagnosis.

Clinically there is tenderness at the middle of the shaft involved and pain is evoked by flexion or extension of the toes. Pain subsides with rest and non-weight bearing and recurs with exertion. Repeated weight bearing causes swelling and redness at the fracture site. When the history fails to elicit trauma and X-rays fail to reveal a fracture, the first view of the callus on X-ray raises the suspicion of a sarcoma.

Treatment

Treatment of the march fracture is symptomatic as this type of fracture heals spontaneously. If pain is severe, a walking plaster cast applied for four weeks will give relief.

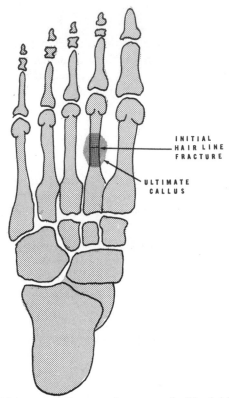

INITIAL
HAIR LINE
FRACTURE

ULTIMATE
CALLUS

FIGURE 82. March fracture of the second metatarsal. The initial fracture is often not observed in routine X-rays or appears as a thin hair-line fracture. Within three weeks, after persistent pain, swelling, and tenderness, the callous formation indicative of healing becomes evident radiologically. This may be the first positive diagnostic sign. Displacement of fragments is rare.

PES CAVUS

Pes cavus, also termed clawfoot, pes arcuatus, or hollow foot (Fig. 83), is a foot with an unusually high arch. The high longitudinal arch causes shortening of the foot and the obliquity of the metatarsals to the floor causes increased pressure on the metatarsal heads with resultant calluses. Due to the high convex arch the extensor ligaments are relatively shortened causing dorsiflexion of the proximal phalanges. The distal phalanges are plantar flexed resulting in clawing of the toes. Calluses form on the dorsum of the toes as well as under the heads. The metatarsophalangeal joints frequently dislocate and the forefoot is usually inflexible.

A very high cavus foot may be totally asymptomatic and symptoms, when they exist, are those of pressure upon the metatarsal heads or unusual

normal forefoot
superimposed

APEX
of
CAVUS

TOES
CLAWED

SHORTENED FOOT

PROMINENT
MET.HEADS

FIGURE 83. Pes cavus. The pes cavus foot has an exaggerated longitudinal arch with its apex at the naviculocuneiform joint. The foot is shorter than normal, the metatarsal heads are prominent, and the toes clawed. The clawing of the toes is due to contracture of the toe extensors. The distal phalanges are flexed and there are dislocations of the metatarso-phalangeal joints. Slanting the illustration until the floor (dotted line) is horizontal depicts the superimposed normal foot.

fatigue when walking or standing. Mildly symptomatic pes cavus is treated with properly fitted shoes with a low heel and a metatarsal bar (Fig. 77). Exercises to stretch the toe extensors and distal toe flexors are recommended. Surgery of soft tissues such as a plantar fasciotomy or tendon transplant is usually unsuccessful. Osteotomies to reshape the foot may be required in severe symptomatic cases.

* * *

There are obviously many other causes of foot pain in the adult that cannot be given full discussion in this monograph. They include fractures, dislocations, neoplastic growths, and infections. Each would require specific consideration that is relegated to the numerous texts available to the interested physician.

BIBLIOGRAPHY

Adams, J. C.: Outline of Orthopaedics. The Williams & Wilkins Co., Baltimore, 1964.
Bailey, H.: Demonstrations of Physical Signs in Clinical Surgery, ed. 13. The Williams & Wilkins Co., Baltimore, 1960.

Barnett, C. H., Davies, D. V., and MacConaill, M. A.: Synovial Joints: Their Structure and Mechanics. Charles C Thomas, Springfield, Ill., 1961.

Basmajian, J. V.: Man's Posture. Arch. Phys. Med. 46:26, Jan. 1965.

DuVries, H. L.: Surgery of the Foot. The C. V. Mosby Co., St. Louis, 1965.

Freeman, M. A., Dean, M. R., and Hanham, I. W.: The Etiology and Prevention of Functional Instability of the Foot. J. Bone Joint Surg. 47:678, 1965.

Kaplan, E.: Some Principles of Anatomy and Kinesiology in Stabilizing Operations of the Foot. Clin. Orthop. 34: 7, 1964.

Licht, S.: Therapeutic Exercises. Elizabeth Licht, Publisher, New Haven, 1958.

Milgram, J. E.: Office Measures for Relief of the Painful Foot. J. Bone Joint Surg. 46-A:1096, 1964.

Rubin, G., and Witten, M: The Talar-Tilt Angle and the Fibular Collateral Ligaments: A Method for the Determination of Talar Tilt. J. Bone Joint Surg. 42-A: 311, 1960.

Wilson, J. N.: The Treatment of Deformities of the Foot and Toes. Brit. J. Phys. Med. 17: 4, April 1954.

Zamosky, I.: Shoe Modifications in Lower-Extremity Orthotics. Bull. Prosthetics Research, Dept. Med. and Surg., Veterans Administration, 10:2, Fall 1964.

Zamosky, I., and Licht, S.: Shoes and Their Modifications. In Orthotics Etcetera, Physical Medicine Library, Vol. 9, edited by S. Licht. Elizabeth Licht, Publisher, New Haven, 1966, p. 388.

CHAPTER 6

Painful Abnormalities of the Toes

HALLUX VALGUS

Hallux valgus is the most common painful deformity of the big toe. Pathologically it is a lateral deviation of the proximal phalanx on the first metatarsal. This condition is generally attributed to the forcing of a foot with a short first metatarsal into a shoe with a pointed toe and high heel. In common usage the symptomatic hallux valgus is termed "bunion," and the terms are used interchangeably.

Diagnosis

There are three components to the "bunion complex": (1) the large toe angulates towards the second toe, (2) the medial portion of the first metatarsal head enlarges, (3) and the bursa over the medial aspect of the joint becomes inflamed and thick walled (Fig. 84). This condition is found most frequently in older women who have a broadened forefoot with a flattened transverse arch in a pronated foot. The big toe frequently oversides the second toe (Fig. 85).

Etiological Concepts

There are many concepts regarding the etiology of hallux valgus. Congenital factors may exist that predispose to deformity in later life. The first metatarsal may be shorter and may be in varus as a residual of metatarsus primus varus (Fig. 68) in childhood. The varus of the first metatarsal may be due to obliquity of the first cuneiform bone which changes the angle of the first tarsometatarsal joint (Fig. 86A). The head of the first metatarsal may be more convex than normal and permit the first phalanx to shift laterally (Fig. 86A). Primary or secondary muscular imbalance

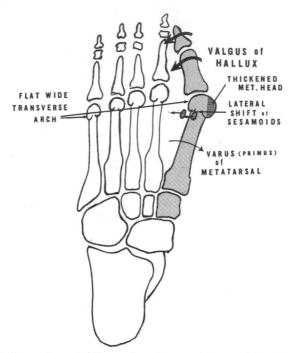

FIGURE 84. Hallux valgus. Hallux valgus is essentially a subluxation of the two phalanges of the big toe in a valgus direction. The first metatarsal deviates in a varus direction and the sesamoids are thus shifted laterally. These major bony and articular changes characterize hallux valgus.

will pull the first phalanx laterally and overcome the ineffectual abductor hallucis (Fig. 86C).

When the foot is forced into a high heeled shoe with a pointed toe and permitted to pronate more from added body weight and debilitation of the intrinsic muscles, the first toe deviates increasingly in a lateral direction. The long tendons of the big toe, both flexor and extensor, shift laterally along with the sesamoid bones and exert traction upon the big toe causing further valgus (Fig. 86B). There are many additional factors contributing to hallux valgus either as primary or secondary influences.

Treatment

Treatment of hallux valgus must be individualized and will depend on the age of the patient, the degree of deformity, and the severity and duration of the symptoms attributed to the hallux valgus. Many patients with severe deformity are symptom free.

If hallux valgus develops before the age of twenty, there is usually a

FIGURE 85. The foot with hallux valgus and bunion. The foot in which hallux valgus predominates is a broad forefoot with a depressed transverse metatarsal arch and a flattened longitudinal arch. The valgus big toe overrides or underlays the second toe which may be secondarily a hammer toe. A swollen inflamed bursa may overlie the enlarged head of the first metatarsal.

family history. In these cases treatment should be conservative and consist of exercises with the wearing of a shoe modified to correct pes planus and pronation (Chapter 4). A stabilizing splint may be worn at night (Fig. 87). A wide shoe with a flat heel should be worn by girls as well as boys. A pouch may be pressed out or cut out at the site of the bunion. If surgery is indicated, the McBride procedure is preferred as it immediately corrects the deformity and eliminates the tendency to recurrence by tendon transplants (Fig. 88). Following surgery the patient must faithfully do corrective exercises and wear proper shoes.

Hallux valgus in the elderly is best treated conservatively including the use of molded shoes which prevent pressure being placed on the protruding portions of the foot. Correction of pronation in the fixed foot of the elderly should be done carefully as the deformities resist alteration. As the hallux valgus deformity of middle age is considered secondary to the strained flattened longitudinal arch and the concomitant splay foot with flattened

101

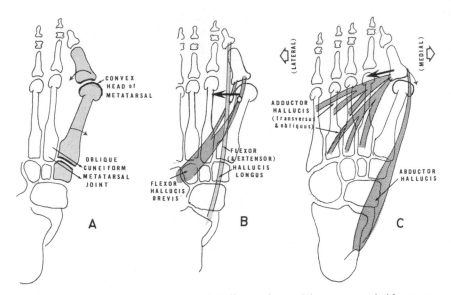

FIGURE 86. Concepts of causation of hallux valgus. The most probable causes held responsible for hallux valgus are: A, excessive convexity of the head of the first metatarsal that permits the phalanx to subluxate laterally. The oblique articular surface of the first cuneiform allows the metatarsal to angle medially to form *metatarsus varus primus*. B, as the phalanges deviate laterally the flexor hallucis brevis and longus tendons on the plantar foot surface and the extensor hallucis longus on the dorsum act like a bowstring. C, imbalance of the foot intrinsics in which the *ad*ductors over pull and shorten. The *ab*ductors are overpowered and elongate.

transverse arch, restoration of these arches may afford relief. Exercise, arch supports, and corrective shoes should always precede surgical intervention. Discussion of the surgical procedures and their merits is beyond the scope of this book. However, two procedures are illustrated in Figure 88 as examples.

HALLUX RIGIDUS

Hallux rigidus is the second most common of the painful problems of the toes. Because of inflexibility of the metatarsophalangeal joint of the big toe, the toe is unable to dorsiflex, which interferes with a smooth takeoff during gait. Every step normally requires extension (dorsiflexion) of the big toe and impairment of motion at this joint may cause pain. A rigid toe that is asymptomatic does not require treatment. Only the partially rigid toe may be symptomatic, and once the fusion is complete, pain may disappear.

FIGURE 87. Night splint for juvenile hallux valgus.

Diagnosis

Usually the patient with hallux rigidus complains of pain elsewhere in the foot resulting from attempts to avoid big toe stress. The patient shifts his weight to the outer border of the foot in order to prevent motion in the big toe. The foot is adducted and inverted to "roll-off" the head of the fifth metatarsal during walking. This is a tiring gait and pressure symptoms occur under the lateral metatarsal heads as well as at the first metatarsophalangeal joint which cannot be completely eliminated in walking.

Treatment

Hallux rigidus requires a shoe with a wide forefoot which permits the forefoot to adduct and that is high enough to permit motion of the entire foot within it. A metatarsal pad placed under the first metatarsal and behind its head raises it and prevents dorsiflexion of the big toe. A metatarsal bar placed outside the shoe with an adequate rocker base aids the gait. A steel plate in the sole prevents flexion deformity of the shoe (Fig. 89).

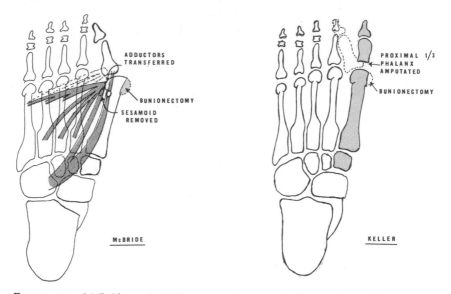

FIGURE 88. McBride and Keller operations for hallux valgus. The McBride operation consists of trimming the bunion, plicating the capsule on the medial aspect of the metatarsal head, and transplanting the adductor conjoined tendon from the base of the proximal phalanx to the outer head of the metatarsal. The adductor group now pulls the metatarsal laterally and does not subluxate the phalanx. The Keller operation trims the bunion and amputates the proximal one third of the proximal phalanx. The muscular attachments to the phalanx are removed. The sesamoids retract and the big toe shortens.

Surgery for hallux rigidus usually consists of resection of the joint and remodeling of the metatarsal head.

HAMMER TOES

Diagnosis

Hammer toe is a fixed flexion deformity of the interphalangeal joint. Any toe may be affected, but it is more prevalent in the second toe. In this condition there is dorsiflexion of the proximal phalanx and flexion of the distal and middle phalanges (Fig. 90). The distal phalanx may point straight ahead but usually points downward. Calluses may form at its tip and also on the dorsum of the flexed interphalangeal joints from pressure against the shoe.

If the hammer toe is severe, the proximal phalanx will frequently sublux. The capsules and tendons on the flexed surfaces become contracted while on the opposite side they stretch. If there is a flexion deformity of only the distal phalanx, the condition is known as "mallet toe."

104

FIGURE 89. Hallux rigidus. Due to damage of the metatarsophalangeal joint, which becomes rigid, the toe will not flex on toe-off of the gait, and pain can occur at each step. Treatment consists of preventing stress on the rigid toe by placing a steel plate in the shoe sole to prevent bending and a rocker bar to permit pain free gait.

Hammer toes are occasionally congenital in which case they occur in more than one toe and are associated with other congenital foot deformities. The acquired variety is the most common and usually occurs in a pronated foot. New shoes which are too short will often cause toes to hammer as will tight elastic stockings of the wrong size. The second toe frequently becomes hammered in the hallux valgus as the big toe encroaches upon and under the second toe (Fig. 85). Hammer toes may follow surgery done for hallux valgus or hallux rigidus in which the flexor tendons are cut.

Treatment

In the treatment of hammer toes it is important to avoid pressure over the protruding joints by the use of properly fitting shoes. The protruding

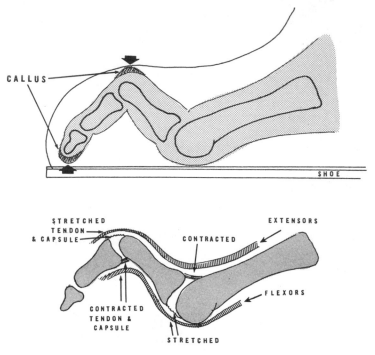

FIGURE 90. Hammer toe. The hammer toe is most often a flexion deformity of the interphalangeal joint with the capsule and tendons contracted on the concave surface. Subluxation is frequent. The proximal phalanx is usually extended and the distal phalanx flexed and flexible. Pressure and friction result in painful calluses forming.

joints may be protected by properly cut and fitted pads or by bulging or cutting the shoe away from the potential callous site. The bulge in the shoe is made with a shoemaker's swan. The severely deformed foot may require custom-made "space shoes."

Manually stretching the contracted tissues of the flexed toes is seldom effective. When the deformity is disabling, surgery to fuse the toes in a straight position may be indicated. In the young, before changes become irreversible, tendon transplants are advocated. This consists of transplanting the flexor tendons to the extensor side of the toes. This procedure is feasible only in the middle three toes because transplanting tendons on the big toe will cause it to rotate and will result in a deformity as troublesome as the hammer toe.

Parents of very young children often express concern over a toe that overrides its neighbor. The fifth toe usually overrides the fourth. It is best to leave this condition untreated other than insuring proper shoes. If the condition becomes symptomatic, tenotomies and capsulotomies may be beneficial. The practice of amputating the fifth toe is usually rejected by the family.

106

BIBLIOGRAPHY

Adams, J. C.: Outline of Orthopaedics, ed. 5. The Williams & Wilkins Co., Baltimore, 1964.

Chomeley, J. A.: Hallux Valgus in Adolescents. Proc. Roy. Soc. Med. 51:903, 1958.

DuVries, H. L.: Surgery of the Foot. The C. V. Mosby Co., St. Louis, 1965.

Kelikian, H.: Hallux Valgus and Allied Deformities of the Forefoot and Metatarsalgia. W. B. Saunders Co., Philadelphia, 1965, pp. 4-17.

Keller, W. L.: Surgical Treatment of Bunions and Hallux Valgus. New York Med. J. 80:741, 1904.

Lapidus, P. W.: Operation for Correction of Hammer Toe. J. Bone Joint Surg. 21:4, 1939.

Lewin, P.: The Foot and Ankle: Their Injuries, Diseases, Deformities and Disabilities, ed. 4. Lea & Febiger, Philadelphia, 1959.

McBride, E. D.: A Conservaitve Operation for Bunions. J. Bone Joint Surg. 10:735, 1928.

Mikhail, I. K.: Bunion, Hallux Valgus, and Metarsus Primus Varus. Surg. Gynec. Obstet. 111:637, 1960.

Milgram, J. E.: Office Procedures for Relief of the Painful Foot. J. Bone Joint Surg. 46-A:1095, 1964.

Taylor, R. G.: The Treatment of Claw Toes by Multiple Transfers of Flexor into Extensor Tendons. J. Bone Joint Surg. 33-B539, 1951.

Wilson, J. N.: The Treatment of Deformities of the Foot and Toes. Brit. J. Phy. Med. 17:73, April 1954.

Wilson, J. N.: V-Y Correction for Varus Deformity of the Fifth Toe. Brit. J. Surg. 41:133, 1953.

Zamosky, I., and Licht, S.: Shoes and Their Modifications. In Orthotics Etcetera, Physical Medicine Library, Vol. 9, edited by S. Licht. Elizabeth Licht, Publisher, New Haven, 1966, p 388.

CHAPTER 7

Painful Conditions of the Heel

There are many varied reasons for a painful heel which can be classified under three headings: (1) pain arising in tissues behind and under the heel, (2) pain arising within the bones and joints of the heel, and (3) pain arising from a source not in the heel but referred there.

PLANTAR FASCIITIS

Pain felt *under the heel* is most frequently caused by a plantar fasciitis occurring with or without a "calcaneal spur." It is common in occupations which entail excessive standing or walking especially when the patient has been unaccustomed to such activity. It is more common in a pronated foot which has a flattened longitudinal arch and frequently occurs after a period of bed rest. Males are more susceptible.

A bony prominence or spur may develop at the attachment of the plantar fascia to the calcaneus. This bony prominence may extend transversely across the entire plantar surface of the bone and is considered an ossification and calcification resulting from traction of the plantar fascia upon the periosteum and occurs commonly without pain.

Pain and tenderness beneath the anterior portion of the heel often radiating into the sole is the presenting complaint. Examination reveals a point of deep tenderness at the anterior medial area of the calcaneus, the point of attachment of the plantar fascia (Fig. 91). X-rays reveal nothing or a typical spur coming forward from the calcaneus. A spur is probably a coincidental finding as they are often found in asymptomatic feet and often not found in patients with symptoms. The pain may be attributed to an infracalcaneal bursitis under the fascial attachment, to a traumatic periostitis, or the tearing of some of the fibers attaching to the bone.

Treatment is directed towards alleviating the pressure of weight bearing. Raising the heel ¼ in. removes the tension placed on the calcaneus by the Achilles tendon and releases the tension of the fascia by plantar

FIGURE 91. Sites of pain in the region of the heel.

flexing the forefoot. A sponge rubber cushion with its center removed may be placed under the heel or a hole may be drilled into the sole of the shoe at the site of the heel and covered with sponge rubber (Fig. 92).

Injections of cortisone and Novocain into the painful region are effective. They may be injected directly into the area through the heel pad or by entering the heel from either the medial or lateral approach (Fig. 93). The injection is given at the site of maximum tenderness, and it is rarely necessary to give more than three weekly injections for relief. Any of the above measures may be used singly or in combination. It is rare that surgical removal of the spur and stripping of the plantar fascia from its posterior attachment must be resorted to. A high incidence of recurrence after surgery is claimed by many and denied by some.

PAINFUL HEEL PAD

Instead of localized pain as in plantar fasciitis, the pain may be generalized over the entire calcaneal pad. This pad is composed of fatty tissue and elastic fibrous tissue enclosed within compartments formed by fibrous septa. Young tissue has an elasticity which acts as a "shock absorber," but the elasticity decreases with age and the weight of the body must be borne by the unpadded calcaneus. This causes pain and if the condition is untreated, it results in scar formation and calcification of the calcaneus. Acute stress upon the pad may rupture or strain the compartments and cause temporary loss of compressibility.

The usual painful heel pad is self-limited and responds to relieving the pressure by either inserting a sponge rubber heel pad as described in treat-

FIGURE 92. Shoe modification in treatment of the calcaneal spur. The lining of the insole is removed and a hole is drilled into the heel. The site of maximum tenderness of the heel determines where the hole should be drilled. A sponge rubber pad covers the hole.

ment of the spur or by raising the heel to transfer the weight anteriorly. Infiltration of 5 to 10 cc. of Novocain under the pad may relieve the symptoms.

DUPUYTREN'S CONTRACTURE

Dupuytren's contracture, similar to that found in the palm, may occur in the plantar fascia (Fig. 91). This condition presents lobulated firm nodules that appear to coalesce within the plantar fascia. They usually occur in middle age and apparently occur more frequently in patients with epilepsy.

The tumors are fibrous and biopsy reveals cellular components of proliferating fibroblasts that may be confused with fibrosarcoma. They are adherent to the skin but show no signs of inflammation. They grow slowly and their symptoms are those of a mechanical nature. Treatment consists of

FIGURE 93. Injection technique in plantar fasciitis. The point of maximum tenderness of the plantar fascia can be injected directly through the heel pad. This is the area where the fascia inserts into the calcaneus. The site can be reached from the lateral or medial approach but localization by this approach is less accurate.

excision of the entire mass and the involved fascia. As in the similar palmar lesions, recurrences are frequent but the condition is benign.

ACHILLES PARATENDINITIS

Inflammation of the paratendinous tissues may cause pain on the posterior aspect of the heel in the region of the Achilles tendon insertion (Fig. 91). The term tenosynovitis is a misnomer when applied to this condition as the Achilles tendon has no synovial tendon sheath. The inflammation occurs in the loose connective tissue about the tendon known as paratenon.

Trauma or stress is usually the cause. There is generalized tenderness when the tendon is squeezed by the examiner's fingers. The tendon usually appears normal but there may be some thickening. Occasionally it is swollen, distended, and exhibits crepitation during motion. Running, jumping, or dancing which stretches the Achilles tendon causes pain.

Treatment consists of immobilization of the ankle in a below-the-knee plaster cast for four weeks. Cortisone injected deep to the tendon may be beneficial. This injection may enter the inflamed retrocalcaneal bursa which may be the cause of the painful Achilles tendon. Surgical excision of the inflamed connective tissues or the inflamed bursa may be needed.

POSTERIOR CALCANEAL BURSITIS

Pain and tenderness of the posterior aspect of the heel and under the skin occurring especially in women is due to a postcalcaneal bursitis which is inflammation of the bursa located between the Achilles tendon and the skin (Fig. 91). The condition is usually caused by friction from ill-fitting shoes and is prevalent in women who wear high heels. The bursa is usually visibly inflamed and often distended with fluid. Chronic irritation will thicken the walls of the bursa and the overlying skin.

Examination reveals an inflamed and thickened area at the back of the heel where the upper margin of the shoe rubs and tenderness and swelling are easily detected. Treatment begins with properly fitted shoes with moderately low heels. Moleskin placed over the thickened skin prevents further friction. The backs of the shoes may have to be cut out or the heel raised inside the shoe. Surgical excision of the bursa is never indicated. Drainage of the swollen bursa may be done by needle aspiration followed by the insertion of hydrocortisone into the sac.

CALCANEAL APOPHYSITIS

Calcaneal apophysitis, also called Sever's disease, is a painful condition occurring in adolescents. Most prevalent in active adolescent boys between the ages of 8 and 13 years, it is the result of an acute or chronic strain of the Achilles tendon on the posterior apophysis of the calcaneus which has not yet fused. It has been classified among the general osteochondroses syndromes which include Calvé-Legg-Perthes disease of the hip and Osgood-Schlatter disease of the tibial tuberosity and can be considered a traction injury.

A diagnosis of apophysitis is suggested when a teen-ager complains of pain and sensitivity at the back of the heel below the attachment of the Achilles tendon. The condition is often bilateral. Walking may be completely pain free, and often the only complaint is tenderness to touch or pressure. As wearing shoes may cause pain, there may be some swelling in the area. The pain is aggravated by standing on tiptoes or running.

X-rays are usually of no assistance in diagnosis. The noted "fragmentation" of the apophysis does not significantly differ from that of the normal heel at that age, but unilateral fragmentation with bony condensation of the epiphysis does supplement the clinical picture and confirms the diagnosis.

Treatment is symptomatic. The condition is self-limited, and symptoms usually subside spontaneously. Efforts should be made to curtail the physical activities of the child to within the limits of his pain until symptoms subside. This presents a problem in active boys as symptoms may persist for many months if trauma continues. A shoe heel built up ¼ in. places the foot in equinus and lessens the strain of the Achilles at its insertion. Crutches may be beneficial when the condition is unilateral. In severe cases the leg is placed in a plaster cast extending above the knee; the knee is flexed and the foot placed in equinus. The prognosis of ultimate recovery without residual disability allays parental concern when pain and tenderness persist.

RUPTURED ACHILLES TENDON

A partial or complete rupture of the Achilles tendon may occur at the narrowest portion of the tendon some 2 in. above its point of attachment. It occurs most often in men between 40 and 50 years of age and has its highest incidence in men with normally sedentary habits who suddenly engage in more violent activities.

Rupture of the Achilles tendon occurs in several manners: (1) an extra stretch to a fully stretched tendon, (2) forceful ankle dorsiflexion when the ankle is relaxed and unprepared, or (3) direct trauma to the tendon while it is taut.

The major complaint is acute agonizing pain felt in the lower calf which makes walking impossible. The patient's feet are examined while he is kneeling on a table with his feet hanging over the edge. In this position the affected foot is less plantar flexed than the other if rupture is complete. A gap in the Achilles tendon can often be palpated and the belly of the gastrocnemius is retracted into the upper calf (Fig. 94). If rupture is complete, the ankle can be dorsiflexed to a greater degree than normal, but if the rupture is partial, dorsiflexion is not increased. The *Simmond's test* consists of squeezing the calf while patient is lying prone with both feet over the edge of the examining table. In the normal ankle, gastroc plantar flexion will occur, but in the complete tendon tear the ankle will not move. The patient who has sustained a complete tear cannot rise on his toes. Ecchymoses are found around the heel.

Partial tears usually become complete at a later date. This later tear may be painless with the patient merely experiencing a sudden fall to the ground

RETRACTED
CALF MUSCLE

NORMAL
TENDO ACHILLIS

TORN TENDON

FIGURE 94. Torn Achilles tendon. Most Achilles tendon tears are complete and occur approximately two inches above the calcaneal insert. The calf muscle retracts towards the popliteal space and a "gap" often can be felt at the site of the tear. Patient cannot rise on his toes.

as his leg "gives out" as if he had been tripped. Examination will confirm the complete tear.

Achilles tendon tears require early surgical treatment. A two month lapse after the tear decreases the possibility of success although repairs after one year have been successful. The surgically repaired tendon is immobilized for approximately four weeks in plaster to allow healing. This is followed by a gradual exercise program to strengthen the calf muscle.

SUBTALAR ARTHRITIS

Pain that is felt *within the heel* may be *referred* from an arthritic subtalar joint (Fig. 91). Arthritis of this joint frequently follows trauma, such as a fracture of the calcaneus. Pain is felt on motion of the subtalar joint, and X-rays reveal irregularity of the bones between the talus and the calcaneus. Crepitation may be elicited by this motion, and tenderness may be elicited from pressure over the sinus tarsi in front of the lateral malleolus. Muscle spasm, especially of the peroneal group, may exist in an attempt to splint the subtalar joint. Weight bearing is painful and rest affords relief. Conservative treatment is usually unsatisfactory but surgical fusion may be necessary if symptoms warrant.

FRACTURES

A fracture must always be suspected when pain in the heel occurs after trauma. Fracture of the calcaneus may result whenever a falling person lands on his feet. Characteristic signs suggest a fracture (Fig. 95). The heel is broadened, and the hollows beneath the malleoli are obliterated because of exudate. Ecchymosis later appears around the heel. All movements of the calcaneus are painful and markedly restricted. X-rays must be taken to confirm the presence, site, and extent of the fracture.

Fractures of the calcaneus result in prolonged incapacity and in some cases permanent disability and pain. A fracture of the calcaneus may be accompanied by a compression fracture of a vertebra or avulsion of the Achilles tendon from its insertion. These must be kept in mind when dealing with a fractured calcaneus. The treatment of calcaneal fractures is beyond the scope of this book and the reader is referred to the literature on the subject.

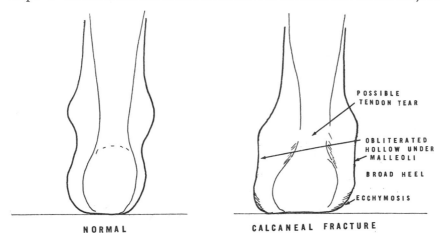

POSSIBLE
TENDON TEAR

OBLITERATED
HOLLOW UNDER
MALLEOLI

BROAD HEEL

ECCHYMOSIS

NORMAL

CALCANEAL FRACTURE

FIGURE 95. Fracture of the calcaneus. A fracture of the calcaneus is suspect when there is a history of trauma and the heel appears broad, the hollows below the malleoli are obliterated, and there is ecchymosis in the plantar surface of the heel. Motion is restricted in attempting inversion and eversion of the calcaneus. Gait is painful. X-rays confirm the diagnosis.

REFERRED PAIN

Pain can be referred to the region of the heel from entrapment of the posterior tibial nerve and its calcaneal branch. This condition is fully discussed in Chapter 9 and depicted in Figure 105. Pain may be referred to the region of the heel from irritation of the S_1 nerve root in lumbar discogenic disease (Fig. 108). For no known reason pain in the heel is a frequent complaint in a patient with early rheumatoid spondylitis.

BIBLIOGRAPHY

Adams, J. C.: Outline of Orthopaedics, ed. 5. The Williams & Wilkins Co., Baltimore, 1964.

DuVries, H. L.: Surgery of the Foot. The C. V. Mosby Co., St. Louis, 1965.

Gross, D.: Ankylosing Spondylitis. Folia Rheumat. 1, Documenta Geigy, Basel, Switzerland, 1965.

Hooker, C. H.: Rupture of the Tendo Calcaneus. J. Bone Joint Surg. 45-B:360, 1963.

Lindholm, A.: A New Method of Operation in Subcutaneous Rupture of the Achilles Tendon. Acta Chir. Scand. 117:261, 1959.

Meyerding, H., and Shellito, J. G.: Dupuytren's Contracture of the Foot. J. Int. Coll. Surg. 11:596, 1948.

Moseley, H. F.: Traumatic Disorders of the Ankle and Foot. Clin. Sympos. 17-3:30, 1965.

Turek, S. L.: Orthopaedics: Principles and Their Application. J. B. Lippincott, Philadelphia, 1959.

Watson-Jones, R.: Fractures and Joint Injuries, ed. 4. The Williams & Wilkins Co., Baltimore, 1955.

Wilson, J. N.: The Treatment of Deformities of the Foot and Toes. Brit. J. Phys. Med. 17:73, April 1954.

CHAPTER 8

Injuries to the Ankle

The sprained ankle is the most common injury that causes pain in the ankle. This condition varies from a simple strain of the ligaments to tearing of the ligaments with or without avulsion of the bones to which they attach. The most severe injury is the fracture-dislocation. The unwary physician who diagnoses every injury to the ankle as a "mere sprain" is harboring a false sense of security and denying proper treatment to his patient. The statement of Watson-Jones that "it is worse to sprain an ankle than to break it" has foundation if every sprain receives the same diagnosis and treatment.

The ankle joint is between the talus, tibia, and fibula and is stable because of its mechanical configuration and ligamentous supports (Figs. 3 and 4). The talus has no muscles attached to it, fits snugly between the two malleoli, and is directly aligned below the tibia. In the dorsiflexed position the broader aspect of the talus is forced between the malleoli, and no lateral motion is permitted. In the plantar flexed position the narrow portion of the talus presents itself between the malleoli and some lateral motion is possible (Fig. 5). The neutral position and especially the plantar flexed position therefore lend themselves the most to the possibility of a sprain.

The lateral and medial collateral ligaments stabilize the ankle joint yet permit plantar and dorsiflexion (Fig. 6). The medial ligaments have an eccentric axis of rotation (Fig. 7) so that all are taut in the neutral position, but the posterior strands relax in plantar flexion and the anterior fibers relax in dorsiflexion. The lateral collateral ligaments have a central axis and remain taut in all ranges of plantar or dorsiflexion.

The ligaments run from the malleoli to the talus, calcaneus, and the navicular. They are supplied with sensory nerves which, when stretched, invoke a reflex muscle spasm which protects the joint from further motion.

The ankle suffers a "sprain" when the ligaments are overstretched. This occurs most frequently when a stress is applied to the ankle that is in an unstable position. The ankle is most unstable when plantar flexed, and it is in this position that forceful inversion or eversion will stretch the ligaments. This action can occur when running, walking over uneven ground, in athletic activities, or even from unaccustomed walking in high heels.

The word "sprain" (Latin: *exprimere:* to "press out") is literally defined as "a joint injury in which some of the fibers of a supporting ligament are ruptured but the continuity of the ligament remains intact," * without dislocation or fracture. This definition taken literally leaves many ambiguous concepts and gives little basis for proper treatment.

INVERSION SPRAINS

The commonest sprain occurs from inversion stress when the foot is slightly plantar flexed and results in stretch of the lateral collateral ligaments. The anterior talofibular ligament is the most commonly affected. If the inversion stress occurs with the ankle at right angle, the calcaneofibular ligament receives the stretch force.

Strain is merely an overstretching of the ligament without disruption of the integrity of its fibers or avulsion from its bony attachment. This may be considered a minor injury and recovery occurs within a few weeks. If the stress is more severe, the fibers may tear and a severe *sprain* has occurred. The ligament rarely tears in its middle but sustains a tear at its proximal or distal point of attachment. A small fragment of bone may be avulsed with the ligament rather than the ligament itself being torn.

The simple strain retains normal joint stability, whereas the severe sprain with tear of the ligament or avulsion of its bony attachment results in instability. The ankle joint dislocates. The degree of dislocation termed *subluxation* implies partial separation of the bones with large areas remaining in contact, whereas *dislocation* connotes complete separation of the adjacent bones. The differentiation of simple strain from a sprain with some degree of dislocation is suspected clinically and verified by X-ray.

Diagnosis

The diagnosis of the injury is best made at the site of the accident when the patient has a clear recollection of the manner of injury. Later the details become vague and the site of pain is less localized. The subsequent swelling and ecchymosis also are less specific at the later date. The history given by the patient or a bystander will reveal the ankle motion that caused the injury and the site of immediate pain and tenderness. There may have been an audible "snap" or a sensation of "tearing."

---

* Dorland's Illustrated Medical Dictionary, ed 24. W. B. Saunders Co., Philadelphia, 1965.

In the simple strain, if the foot is passively inverted, the talus remains in its proper position and no gap can be palpated between it and the malleolus. Protective spasm may deceive the examiner in the early phase, therefore any severe sprain should be considered to be a potential tear or avulsion until confirmed or denied by X-ray. If a tear has occurred, the foot can be inverted to a greater degree than normal and the talus separates from the lateral malleolus. A palpable sulcus may permit insertion of a finger tip between the talus and the lateral malleolus. X-rays taken with the foot inverted will reveal abnormal tilt of the talus within the mortice (Fig. 96).

All significant ankle injuries should be X-rayed. To reveal tilting of the talus within the mortice, which normally is insignificant, the ankle must be fully inverted, then X-rayed in this position. The practice of injecting Novocain into the area of ligamentous strain to "overcome" the pain and spasm is usually unnecessary if the ankle is moved gently and slowly. The degree of talar tilt indicates the presence and extent of a tear of the ligaments.

With a sprain there will ultimately be an effusion into the ankle joint that will distend the joint and cause the foot to invert and dorsiflex. The swelling is first noted beneath the extensor tendons, usually anterior to the lateral malleolus, and eventually will be seen on either side of the Achilles tendon behind the malleoli. Ecchymosis may occur indicating injury to blood vessels in the area

The range of plantar and dorsiflexion of the ankle joint may remain

FIGURE 96. Lateral ligamentous sprain and avulsion. The lateral ligaments of the ankle are depicted in C. The anterior talofibular and the calcaneofibular ligaments are the ligaments most frequently involved in inversion injuries. A is the simple sprain in which the ligaments remain intact and the talus remains stable within the mortice. B depicts avulsion of the lateral ligaments, and the talus becomes unstable and *tilts* within the mortice when the calcaneus is adducted.

normal in spite of severe lateral ligamentous tear. Normally inversion and eversion is markedly limited or nonexistent in the dorsiflexed joint so any such motion that occurs with the foot dorsiflexed indicates ligamentous laxity or tear. To test this motion the calcaneus must be grasped and motion attempted there. A false impression will be received if the forefoot rather than the calcaneus is moved. *Testing for excessive range of motion should not delay the institution of appropriate treatment.* Specific treatment after establishing a more precise diagnosis will be possible and more effective if immediate care is instituted regardless of the severity of the injury.

Treatment

Control of swelling is the immediate consideration. Effusion and hemorrhage distend the joint and overstretch the ligaments. The presence of effusion also favors the formation of adhesions which delay healing. Swelling can be minimized by (1) the immediate application of a firm bandage, (2) the application of cold, and (3) elevation of the leg. Bandaging must be firm and must include the entire foot from behind the toes to the lower half of the leg. Two inch gauze, crepe bandage, or an elastic bandage may be used. Adhesive tape is permissible but less desirable because it may be irritating to the skin and difficult to remove.

The bandaged ankle should be placed in cold or ice water immediately. If this is not feasible, ice packs around the elevated foot may be used. The duration of immersion is arbitrary and varies with the severity of the injury. As a rule 15 to 20 minutes of immersion, followed by elevating the leg, repeated every 3 to 6 hours, will suffice. Oral phenylbutazone may be used in the hope of minimizing inflammation.

X-rays should be taken as soon as possible especially if fracture is suspected. Routine films through the bandage will reveal the more obvious fractures. If avulsion of the ligaments is suspected, as it should in all severe injuries, "stress" X-rays should be taken. The attending physician should hold the foot in marked inversion while the films are taken to insure that proper views are taken.

If only a strain is diagnosed, the foot may be rebandaged daily and ice packs continued for several more days. After three or four days the ice packs are replaced by hot soaks. The bandage should not be removed too soon or the swelling may return. Usually after seven to ten days the bandage can be removed safely.

Non-weight-bearing exercises should be started within the first few days. They should be done actively by the patient and not forcefully by a therapist or a relative. The foot should be moved through full range of motion: full plantarflexion, dorsiflexion, inversion and eversion, and toe flexion.

These motions done frequently during the day will help disperse the edema and avoid the formation of adhesions as well as maintain muscle tone. Hot and cold contrast baths, whirlpool, ultrasound therapy, and iontophoresis, if available, may hasten recovery but are not superior to heat and active exercises.

When the swelling has significantly subsided or disappeared and the ankle has been proven to have no ligamentous tear, the ankle should be taped in a basket weave fashion (Fig. 97) and weight bearing resumed. Competitive sports should be avoided for at least one to three weeks depending on the appearance, function, and pain of the ankle. If discomfort persists and the patient feels insecure in spite of the ankle appearing stable in clinical examination and stress X-rays, a lateral wedge may be added to the heel of the shoe (Fig. 98). Taping of the ankle should be continued for several weeks.

Treatment of the inversion injury with avulsion or tear of the lateral ligament must be energetic. A plaster cast is applied holding the foot at a right angle to the leg with the foot and ankle in slight *eversion*. The cast is applied even in the presence of swelling and is removed and replaced as the swelling decreases and the cast becomes loose fitting. The cast should be kept on for ten weeks and may include a walking heel.

Some favor surgical repair of completely avulsed ligaments, but it is

FIGURE 97. Taping a sprained ankle. The purpose of taping an ankle is to prevent further stretching of the injured ligaments until healing has occurred. The ankle must be inverted or everted to place the strained ligament at rest. The center figure depicts an avulsed lateral ligament. The tape here begins from inside and runs under the foot to finish on the outer leg holding the heel *everted*. The horizontal strips minimize rotation of the forefoot.

SINGLE
BAR
BRACE

"T" STRAP

avulsed
ligament

LATERAL
WEDGE

NORMAL
SHOE

SPLAY

"FREE" ANKLE
JOINT

FIGURE 98.　Conservative treatment of the chronic recurrent dislocation of the ankle joint. When the lateral ligaments are avulsed and improperly treated the ankle becomes unstable. A lateral heel and sole wedge plus a splay heel maintains the foot in an everted position. An inside single bar brace with an inside pulling "T" strap maintains eversion.

generally accepted that an ankle properly immobilized for a sufficient length of time will heal satisfactorily. After removal of the cast, active exercises should be initiated in order to regain range of motion and strength of the foot and ankle muscles. The proprioceptive sense of the ligaments and muscles must be retrained by coordination and balancing exercises.

"Chronic sprain" or recurrent dislocations usually imply improper treatment of the initial acute injury. Treatment of these recurring sprains must include support of the ankle. This is done by using an outside heel and sole wedge, a "splay" heel on the shoe, a brace with a "T" strap pulling the ankle towards the inside upright bar, exercises to strengthen the evertor muscles of the foot and ankle, and exercises to improve balance coordination. Persistence of disability will often require surgical intervention.

EVERSION SPRAINS

An injury to the ankle that forcefully *everts* the ankle will usually cause bony damage rather than straining or tearing of the medial ligament alone as in the *inversion* type of injury. The more frequent ankle injury, forceful inversion, causes mostly ligamentous injury and only rarely involves bone. In an eversion injury the medial ligament is so strong that fracture or avulsion of the tibia will occur before the ligament tears. Although tearing of the deltoid ligament is infrequent it must be constantly suspected to prevent the serious consequences of improper treatment.

Tibiofibular Ligament Tear

A sprain of the medial ligaments may tear the inferior tibiofibular ligament. This ligamentous tear permits the ankle mortice to widen and causes an unstable ankle joint. The talus is allowed lateral motion within the mortice which ultimately leads to degenerative changes of the joint (Fig. 99).

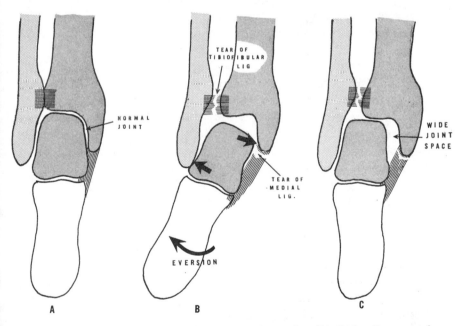

FIGURE 99. Avulsion of medial ligament and anterior tibiofibular ligaments from eversion injury to the ankle. A depicts the normal ankle mortice with the talus snugly between the malleoli. The eversion stress separates the malleoli (*arrows*), tears the anterior tibiofibular ligaments and the medial deltoid ligament, B. Once the ankle has returned to its neutral position, C, a wide space remains between the talus and the medial malleolus which is a diagnostic sign on X-ray. With the wide mortice the ankle remains unstable.

Diagnosis

Widening of the ankle mortice can easily be missed clinically. The tear of the tibiofibular ligament and the separation of the malleoli must be suspected and confirmed by X-ray studies. The pathognomonic sign on X-ray is a widening of the joint space between the medial border of the talus and the medial malleolus (Fig. 99C). Routine ankle views may fail to reveal this separation as the lower tibia and fibula frequently overlap on a direct anterior-posterior view. An oblique view when compared with a similar view of the other ankle will often reveal the separation.

Treatment

Treatment of the torn deltoid and inferior tibiofibular ligaments attempts approximating the two malleoli in order to reform the mortice and seat the talus snugly. This is done by plaster casting with the ankle compressed bilaterally. After ten days, or sooner if the swelling has subsided and the cast has loosened, a new cast is applied. After three to six weeks a third cast is applied to further compress the malleoli together. No weight bearing is permitted for eight weeks.

Internal fixation with a screw inserted between the tibia and the fibula may be necessary to reduce the separation and approximate the two fragments. Many feel this procedure is always indicated, but *internal fixation with a screw does not permit earlier weight bearing, nor does it eliminate the need for plaster casting.* The screw merely assures anatomical reduction and immobilization within the cast. It presents all the adverse effects of open reduction as opposed to closed reduction.

FRACTURES AND FRACTURE DISLOCATIONS

Treatment of fractures and fracture dislocations is beyond the scope of this book. Fractures and fracture dislocations result from stresses similar to those that cause ligamentous injuries which reaffirms the need for X-ray studies of the injured ankle. Initial treatment of the injured ankle with a possible fracture is as for the severe sprain and involves careful handling to attempt gentle correction of the gross deformity to prevent compounding the fracture and impairing the circulation. Splinting for transportation, elevation of the leg, application of cold, and firm dressing will minimize the swelling without impairment of circulation. The particular fracture must then receive its specific treatment (Fig. 100).

FIGURE 100.   Sites of fracture and ligamentous avulsion. Fractures can occur at
all the depicted sites. These fractures can be single, in combination, with or without
ligamentous tear or avulsion, and with any combination of dislocation. F indicates
fracture, A, avulsion of ligament. Proper diagnosis is by X-ray.

BIBLIOGRAPHY

Clayton, M. L., and Weir, G. J.: Experimental Investigations of Ligamentous
   Healing. Am. J. Surg. 98:373, 1959.
DePalma, A. F.: Section I, Symposium: Injuries to the Ankle Joint. Clin. Orthop.
   Related Res. 42:2, 1965.
DuVries, H. L.: Surgery of the Foot. The C. V. Mosby Co., St. Louis, 1965.
Freeman, M. A. R., Dean, M. R. E., and Hanham, I. W. F.: The Etiology and Pre-
   vention of Functional Instability of the Foot. J. Bone Joint Surg. 47-B:678.
Griffiths, J. C.: Tendon Injuries Around the Ankle. J. Joint Surg. 47-B:686.
Kaplan, E.: Some Principles of Anatomy and Kinesiology in Stabilizing Operations
   of the Foot. Clin. Orthop. 34:7, 1964.
Lewin, P.: The Foot and Ankle, ed. 4. Lea & Febiger, Philadelphia, 1959.
McLaughton, H. L.: Trauma. W. B. Saunders Co., Philadelphia, 1959.
Mosely, H. F.: Traumatic Disorders of the Ankle and Foot. Clin. Sympos. 17-3:30,
   1965.
Rubin, G., and Witten, M.: The Talar Tilt Angle and the Fibular Collateral Liga-
   ments. J. Bone Joint Surg. 42-A:311, 1960.

CHAPTER 9

Neurological Disorders of the Foot

Foot disturbances attributable to nerve involvement are rarely due to intrinsic causes in the foot proper. Most neurological disorders of the foot are caused by impairment of nerves proximal to it, involving either a peripheral nerve or some portion of the central nervous system.

INNERVATION OF THE FOOT

The foot and ankle are innervated by spinal segments of L_4, L_5, S_1, and S_2. These segments descend the posterior thigh in the sciatic nerve and ultimately divide into the tibial and the peroneal nerves (Fig. 26) which supply the musculature of the foot and ankle. The muscles which plantar flex the foot and ankle are innervated by the tibial nerve, those that dorsiflex by the deep peroneal branch of the common peroneal nerve, and those that evert by the superficial branch of the common peroneal. The small plantar muscles receive their innervation from the distal branches of the posterior tibial nerve after it has reached the sole of the foot and divided into the lateral and medial plantar nerves.

If the sciatic nerve is severed, total paralysis of all the muscles below the knee will result, together with loss of sensation on the outer side of the leg and almost the whole foot. A small area on the inner surface of the heel will be spared loss of sensation.

The sensory pattern of the peripheral nerves of the leg is shown in Figure 27. The combination of specific motor weakness with hypalgesia of skin surfaces will reveal which nerve or nerves are impaired.

Injury to the deep peroneal nerve impairs dorsiflexion of the foot and toes and causes a drop foot resulting in a steppage gait. Hypalgesia is confined to a small area of the dorsum of the foot between the first and second toes. Because the superficial peroneal nerve remains intact, the foot everts during gait resulting in a valgus foot.

Injury to the superficial peroneal nerve paralyzes the evertors of the foot causing inversion with an ultimate equinovarus foot position. The anterior lateral aspect of the leg and the dorsum of the foot lose sensation. Injury to the common peroneal nerve combines the motor and sensory losses just described for the deep and superficial nerves. The foot is now "dropped" and has some inversion due to the unopposed action of the posterior tibial muscle.

Because the plantar and toe flexors are innervated by the tibial nerve, the patient is unable to rise on his toes or to flex them when this nerve is damaged. There is sensory loss on the plantar surface of the foot with ultimate atrophy of the calf and the intrinsic muscles of the foot. The exact level of nerve injury will determine the extent of motor loss and vice versa.

Determining whether a motor impairment is at (a) the anterior horn cell level, (b) the root level (Fig. 101), (c) the spinal nerve level, or (d) the peripheral nerve level may pose some difficulty. Figure 102 depicts the components leading to the formation of a peripheral nerve and specific muscle innervation. Localization of the site of nerve impairment is possible by manual muscle testing, sensory pattern mapping, and electro-

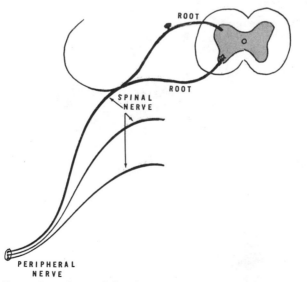

FIGURE 101. Formation of a peripheral nerve. A sensory and motor root emerge from the spinal cord. They merge to form a spinal segmental nerve. The area served by the sensory portion of this nerve is called a dermatome. The muscles innervated by the motor segment are a myotome. Several segmental nerves may merge to form a peripheral nerve which is both sensory and motor.

	L_4	L_5	S_1	S_2
TIBIALIS ANTERIOR — deep peroneal n.	██			
EXTENSOR DIGITORUM LONGUS — deep peroneal n.		██	██	
PERONEUS LONGUS — superficial peroneal n.		██	██	
PERONEUS BREVIS — superficial peroneal n.		██	██	
FLEXOR HALLUCIS LONGUS — posterior tibial n.		██	██	
FLEXOR HALLUCIS BREVIS — posterior tibial n.: plantar br.			██	
EXTENSOR HALLUCIS BREVIS — deep peroneal n.			██	
FLEXOR DIGITORUM LONGUS — posterior tibial n.: plantar br.			██	
EXTENSOR HALLUCIS LONGUS — deep peroneal n.			██	
FLEXOR DIGITORUM BREVIS — posterior tibial n.: plantar br.			██	██
POSTERIOR TIBIALIS — posterior tibial n.			██	██
EXTENSOR DIGITORUM BREVIS — deep peroneal n.			██	██
GASTROCNEMIUS — tibial n.			██	██
SOLEUS — tibial n.				██
SMALL MUSCLES OF SOLE OF FOOT — medial-lateral plantar n.			██	

FIGURE 102. Origin of nerve roots in spinal segments. Chart shows innervation of the muscles involved in gait and the gray area the spinal segments of origin.

myographic testing. More recently nerve conduction determination has entered the field of neuromuscular diagnosis making diagnosis and prognosis more accurate.

The function of any nerve along its path may be impaired by mechanical irritation or compression resulting in an entrapment neuropathy. Here motor and sensory loss and pain may result with the pain usually present at rest and sometimes becoming severe at night. The nerve distal to the site of entrapment is frequently tender. The pain may confuse the examiner by having a retrograde distribution, thus causing suspicion of a peripheral neuropathy arising at a different level.

MORTON'S NEUROMA

Morton's neuroma is an entrapment neuropathy of an interdigital nerve. This is a painful condition resulting from a neuroma, a fusiform swelling about ¾ in. in length, on a digital nerve. It is most commonly found where the interdigital nerve branches into the contiguous aspects of the digits, usually between the third and fourth toes (Fig. 103). An unusual neuroma may be found between the second and third metatarsals.

This condition is found most often in middle-aged women. The pain is neuritic in nature and radiates from a site near the metatarsal heads into the toes. At first, pain occurs only on weight bearing but ultimately occurs even at rest. *Taking the weight off the feet is not as important as removing the shoes.* This desire to remove the shoe and massage and manipulate the foot is indicative of neuroma. Mere rest does not afford relief.

Pressure *between* the metatarsal heads reproduces the pain, whereas metatarsalgia without neuroma causes tenderness *at* the metatarsal heads. Compression of the metatarsal heads together also causes pain in the neuroma. Numbness and hypalgesia of the contiguous aspects of the toes may be elicited and a palpable tumor is frequently found.

Treatment is that of supporting the transverse arch in a suitable broad shoe. Local injection of steroids often gives relief, but surgical excision of the neuroma may ultimately be required.

INTERDIGITAL NEURITIS

Other interdigital nerves may be involved and cause pain. Superficial to the transverse metatarsal ligament, the interdigital nerves pass forward from the sole of the foot to reach the dorsum of the foot. If the toes are hyperextended at the metatarsal joints, the nerves are angulated over the ligament. If there is also some abnormal pressure, a "throbbing" type of

FIGURE 103. Morton's interdigital neuroma. Morton's neuroma is a neurofibroma of the interdigital nerve. The most frequent site is the third branch of the medial plantar nerve as it merges with the lateral plantar nerve to form the digital nerve between the third and fourth toes. Pain occurs in the area and hypalgesia can be elicited in the opposing areas of the toes.

pain is felt in the involved toes. The pain persists after weight bearing and the patient tends to remove his shoe and massage the painful area.

Tenderness can be elicited by pressure *between* the metatarsal heads. This is contrary to metatarsalgia in which the pain occurs mostly during weight bearing and tenderness is elicited by pressure directly upon the metatarsal heads. If the injection of Novocain between the metatarsal heads relieves the pain, the diagnosis of interdigital neuritis is confirmed.

Treatment consists of preventing hyperextension of the toes. Abnormal occupational posture, such as that depicted in Figure 104, must be corrected, and the female patient urged to avoid high heels. A metatarsal pad or bar that flexes the toes may help. Shoes should have adequate width across the metatarsal heads and low heels. If symptoms persist, surgical removal of the neuroma must be considered.

POSTERIOR TIBIAL NERVE ENTRAPMENT

Pain and paresthesia can occur in the plantar aspect of the foot and toes due to an entrapment of the posterior tibial nerve or its plantar branches

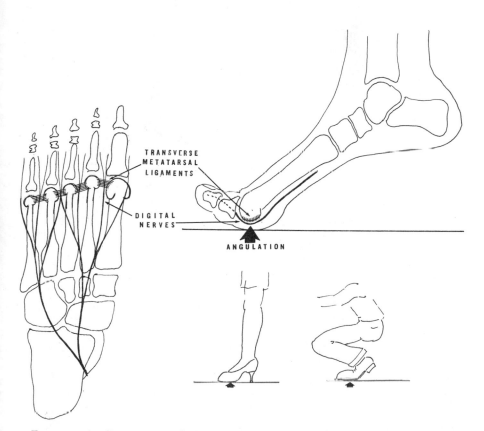

FIGURE 104. Entrapment of the interdigital nerve. The interdigital nerves are sensory to the toes. They come from the plantar nerves in the sole of the foot then pass across the transverse metatarsal ligament to the dorsum of the toes. If they are angulated at the ligament by posture and weight bearing, pain in the foot and numbness of the toes may result.

(Fig. 105). The posterior tibial nerve passes behind and under the medial malleolus beneath the laciniate ligament. It is accompanied by the tendons of the posterior tibial and the flexor digitorum longus and the tibial artery and veins. The laciniate ligament forms a roof over the bony depression behind the medial malleolus converting the area into a tarsal "tunnel."

As the posterior tibial nerve enters the tarsal tunnel, the calcaneal branch emerges above or through the laciniate ligament to supply sensory innervation to the heel. After leaving the tunnel the nerve passes deep to the sole of the foot and divides into a calcaneal branch and the medial and lateral plantar branches. These branches innervate the intrinsic muscles of the foot and supply the sensory branches to the sole. The medial branch carries sensation from the medial three and a half toes and the medial aspect of the sole. The lateral plantar nerve supplies the lateral half of the sole and the other outer toes.

Pressure upon the plantar branches or the posterior tibial nerve within the

FIGURE 105. Entrapment of the posterior tibial nerve and its plantar branches. The posterior tibial nerve passes in a tunnel under the laciniate (talocalcaneal) ligament. It is accompanied by the tendons on the posterior tibial and flexor digitorum longus. The posterior tibial nerve branches into the plantar nerves and gives off a calcaneal branch. The plantar nerves supply the small muscles of the sole and their sensory distribution is shown in figure on the left.

tunnel can occur from trauma such as a fall with the patient landing on his feet, standing on a ladder with soft shoes, acute pronation or acute strain upon a chronically pronated foot which cause impingement of the nerves between the tarsal bones and the sharp edge of the abductor hallucis muscle. Pressure also may occur from an ill-fitting longitudinal arch support that is too high in the arch.

The pain of entrapment of the posterior tibial nerve in the tarsal tunnel is of a "burning" nature and is felt whether standing or at rest. Which of the branches is most affected determines the sensory distribution. If the calcaneal branch is affected, it may mimic the "calcaneal spur" syndrome of the painful heel.

Diagnosis is made by the history and the burning characteristics of the pain in the distribution of the plantar nerve. Tenderness can be elicited over the posterior tibial nerve behind the medial malleolus and the pain frequently can be eliminated by injecting Novocain into the tunnel. Recent studies with nerve conduction determinations have revealed a lengthening of the conduction time in the entrapped nerve. Clinically it is possible to elicit weakness of the toe flexors at the proximal joints, sensory loss, visible wasting of the intrinsics, and a positive Tinel's sign.

Treatment requires postural correction of the foot to alter pronation. When conservative measures fail, surgical decompression of the tunnel may be necessary. When tenosynovitis of the tendons within the tunnel appears to be the cause of compression against the nerve, injection with steroids may be beneficial.

ANTERIOR TIBIAL NEURITIS

Pain can be felt when the deep peroneal nerve is injured on the dorsum of the foot. This nerve (previously called the *anterior tibial* nerve) accompanies the dorsalis pedis artery and becomes superficial below the cruciate crural ligament. At this point there is little tissue protecting the nerve (Fig. 106). It overlies the tarsal bones and is exposed to direct trauma. A poorly designed shoe is often the cause of trauma. Sensory involvement is at the dorsal cleft between the first and second toes. Some weakness of the big toe extensor may be elicited. There may be tenderness over the nerve which can be diagnostically relieved by an injection of Novocain.

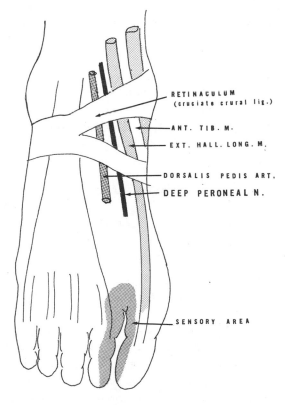

FIGURE 106. Trauma to the deep peroneal nerve. The deep peroneal nerve becomes superficial as it emerges below the cruciate crural ligament. There it is vulnerable to trauma causing pain and numbness in the area shown in the diagram.

COMMON PERONEAL NERVE PALSY

Injury to the common peroneal nerve as it curves around the neck of the fibula will result in weakness of the evertors and dorsiflexors of the foot and cause hypalgesia on the lateral aspect of the leg and the dorsal aspect of the foot. Pain can be elicited by forcefully placing the foot into plantar flexion and inversion which stretches the peroneal nerve. Tenderness can frequently be elicited at the fibular neck and procaine infiltration there may relieve symptoms.

REFERRED NEURITIC PAIN

The nerve roots which make up the sciatic nerve may be injured causing neurological signs in the foot and ankle. The most common cause of this is irritation from a herniated lumbar disk. The exact location of the disk involved is depicted in Figure 107. The dermatome deficiency indicates the nerve root involved (Fig. 108). This, in association with specific motor function (Fig. 102) loss and reflex changes, will locate the level of spinal involvement.

The diagnosis is made by a history of pain, usually in the low back, with radiation down the posterior aspect of the leg into the calf, ankle, even the toes. It is worse on straining at stool. Examination finds limited low back flexibility, paraspinous spasm causing functional scoliosis, and a positive straight leg raising test on the involved side.

SPASTIC PARALYSIS

The foot is involved in spastic conditions resulting from upper motor neuron lesions. In the young, the cause of this is usually cerebral palsy and in the adult a cerebrovascular accident. The findings of hyperactive deep tendon reflexes, spasticity, clonus, and positive Babinski signs reveal the neurological causes. The etiology of upper motor neuron lesions is beyond the scope of this book.

The functional abnormality of the foot in the spastic lower extremity is that of equinovarus in which the toes are unable to clear the floor during walking. Because the foot is plantar flexed the patient cannot place his heel on the ground. Treatment seeks to prevent contractures of the Achilles tendon and to strengthen the ankle dorsiflexors and evertors. The Achilles tendon can be stretched by active and passive exercises often with the assistance of braces.

FIGURE 107. Relationship of nerve roots to disk spaces.

Bracing

Excessive plantar flexion can be prevented by the use of a right ankle joint angle stop on a short leg caliper brace (Fig. 109), either single or double bar. A medial "T" strap can be used to pull the ankle towards the bar and thus counteract inversion of the foot. If the foot is flail or has minimal spasticity, a "piano wire" brace may be all that is necessary to overcome the drop foot and thus permit clearance from the floor during gait (Fig. 110). A night brace may be worn to stretch the Achilles tendon by keeping the foot dorsiflexed during sleeping hours (Fig. 111). Certain types of equinovarus or those resistant to exercise and bracing may be helped surgically by Achilles tendon lengthening or by tenotomy of the posterior tibial tendon and tenotomy of the flexor digitorum longus.

FIGURE 108.   Dermatome mapping of lumbar and sacral roots.

CALIPER SINGLE BAR

"T"STRAP

FIGURE 109. Short leg brace with right-angle stop. This short leg brace stops plantar flexion of the foot at a right angle to prevent drop foot or equinus. It may have a single or a double upright bar. The pull of the "T" strap corrects the inversion when connected to an inside bar.

FIGURE 110. Piano-wire dorsiflexion brace. When the gastrocnemius has minimal spasticity or in a flaccid drop foot, the resilient piano wire elevates the anterior portion of the foot so it clears the floor during walking.

FIGURE 111. Achilles tendon stretching night brace. The eccentric ankle joint forces the bar to varying degrees altering the ankle dorsiflexion. The cuff affords counter pressure. In the right lower picture the rotation of the eccentric joint has forced the foot into dorsiflexion.

The valgus foot that may result from these tenotomies is often preferable to the disability caused by severe equinovarus.

BIBLIOGRAPHY

Bovill, E. G.: Diseases of nerves. *In* Surgery of the Foot, by H. L. DuVries. The C. V. Mosby Co., St. Louis, 1965, p. 279

Cailliet, R.: Bracing for Spasticity. *In* Orthotics Etcetera. Physical Medicine Library, Vol. 9, edited by S. Licht. Elizabeth Licht, Publisher, New Haven, 1966, p. 365.

Goodgold, J., Kopell, H. P., and Spielholz, N. I.: The Tarsal-Tunnel Syndrome. Objective Diagnostic Criteria. New Eng. J. Med., 273: 742, 1965.

Haymaker, W., and Woodhall, B.: Peripheral Nerve Injuries: Principles of Diagnosis, ed. 2. W. B. Saunders, Philadelphia, 1959.

Kopell, H. P., and Thompson, W. A. L.: Peripheral Entrapment Neuropathies. The Williams & Wilkins Co., Baltimore, 1963.

Lam, S. J. S.: A Tarsal-Tunnel Syndrome. Lancet. 2:1354, 1962.

Marinacci, A. A.: Clinical Electromyography. San Lucas Press, Los Angeles, 1955.

Oester, Y. T., and Mayer, J. H.: Motor Examination of Peripheral Nerve Injuries. Charles C Thomas Co., Springfield, Ill., 1960.

Perry, J.: Orthopedic Management of the Lower Extremity in the Hemiplegic Patient. J. Am. Phys. Therap. Assn. 46:345, 1966.

Stamp, W.: Bracing in Cerebral Palsy. J. Bone Joint Surg. 44-A: 1457, 1962.

CHAPTER 10

Dermatological Conditions of the Foot

There are a number of painful dermatological conditions of the foot which include plantar warts, calluses, corns, and various forms of "dermatitis." These are all capable of interfering with normal foot mobility and gait.

CALLUS

A callus is a thickening of the skin, either diffuse or circumscribed, in an area exposed to persistent abnormal pressure or friction. Abnormal foot mechanics precede their formation. In conditions where the transverse arches are depressed, weight bearing by the metatarsal heads will lead to the formation of plantar calluses. In the markedly inverted foot, pressure upon the fifth metatarsal head will result in a callus there. If the toes are clawed or hammered, the skin over the protruding interphalangeal joints will develop calluses where it presses against the shoe.

Calluses may be confused with warts but when pared show normal papillary lines running through the hyperkeratotic area. The lines do not deviate. There may be a translucent core that is well demarcated, but there are no blood vessels in the core.

Treatment consists of application of 40 per cent salicyclic acid plaster and a felt pad with the center cut out to prevent further pressure or friction. Ultimate treatment for calluses requires avoidance of the abnormal contact points by the wearing of corrective shoes. Unless the cause of abnormal foot mechanics and the sites of abnormal pressure and friction are discovered and corrected the lesion will recur after treatment.

NEUROVASCULAR CORN

A variant of corns, the neurovascular corn, may pose a diagnostic problem. It appears over a bony prominence and is sharply demarcated. When pared a small blood vessel appears that lies *parallel* to the surface and not vertical as in the case of warts. The neurovascular corn can be very tender and painful. It is best treated by paring followed by the weekly application of 50 to 100 per cent solution of silver nitrate. In between these treatments a 40 per cent salicylic acid plaster is applied.

"SOFT" CORN

A "soft" corn is a hyperkeratotic lesion found *between* the toes. These corns usually occur between the fourth and fifth toes and are most frequently situated in the web. They result from the pressure of opposing toes and occur in a region that is constantly moist which denys them the chance to become cornified. They are best treated by application of 40 per cent salicylic acid plasters and separation of the toes by sponge rubber pads or lamb's wool. Surgical excision is often necessary, and should there be an underlying bone spur promoting corn formation, it too should be surgically removed.

PLANTAR WARTS

Plantar warts differ from calluses and are not necessarily found over bony prominences. They are sharply circumscribed with their edges clearly demarcated from the surrounding skin (Fig. 112). Their center is darker than the surrounding skin and they may have a mosaic appearance. If the surrounding skin is stretched from the "core," a small cleft appears between it and the surrounding skin. Warts are usually tender to squeezing whereas calluses are usually not. Tenderness in calluses is usually in the bony prominences under it.

Plantar warts are simple papillomas considered to be caused by a virus. There are three varieties of plantar warts. The first is the single wart that often appears under a bony prominence and may, at first, be difficult to differentiate from a callus. When the wart is pared the distinct margin becomes apparent, and its surface is *dotted* by *small capillary tips*. The second variety is the "mother-daughter" type in which a large wart is surrounded by several smaller "satellite" warts. The satellite warts have the same characteristics as the center wart but in the early stages may be more vesicular than the keratotic mother. They are usually extremely painful. The third type, the mosaic, appears as granular calluses that are grouped in a mosaic pattern that may extend over the entire metatarsal surface. The individual cores of the mosaic resemble the single wart.

Treatments are numerous. *Surgery is contraindicated for all plantar warts* as the resulting scar may be more painful than the wart, and new warts can

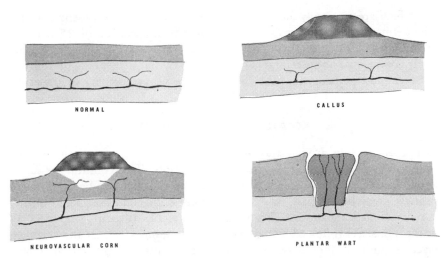

NORMAL

CALLUS

NEUROVASCULAR CORN

PLANTAR WART

FIGURE 112. Dermatological conditions of the foot. The *callus* is merely a hyperkeratotic area that forms at the point of persistent pressure or friction. The *neurovascular corn* is a hyperkeratotic area with an avascular translucent base that may have a blood vessel lying parallel to the surface. *Plantar wart* is a papilloma, cone shaped, with a cleft between it and the surrounding skin. Blood vessels in the *wart* are vertical and the ends are visible when pared.

grow in and along the scar. The objective in treating plantar warts is always to eradicate it with the minimal amount of scarring as the scar may be as painful and disabling as the wart. Application of salicylic acid tape directly to the wart, removed and reapplied several times daily, frequently relieves symptoms in a few days and causes disappearance of the wart in several weeks. They may be curetted and the exposed base cauterized by commercial dry ice, solid carbon dioxide, or liquid nitrogen. Electrocautery may be lightly applied to the base. Plantar warts respond to radiotherapy, but great care must be exercised to protect the surrounding skin with a lead shield.

The mosaic warts may be treated by paring to the point of bleeding then applying 100 per cent silver nitrate to the capillary tips followed by swabbing with a saturated solution of trichloroacetic acid. This is followed by the application of 40 per cent salicylic acid plaster held in place by moleskin for a period of one week. This procedure is repeated weekly until normal skin tissue replaces the wart.

HYPERHIDROSIS

Excessive perspiration, or hyperhidrosis, may be troublesome. It creates or continues dermatological conditions which must be specifically treated but which are adversely affected by hyperhidrosis. In the absence of specific dermatitis, hyperhidrosis can be treated by application of 25 per cent aluminum chloride solution three to four nights each week. There are many commercial antiperspirants on the market that decrease hyperhidrosis but care must be taken that they do not cause skin sensitivity or irritation.

KERATODERMIA PLANTARIS

The entire sole around the margin of the heel may undergo diffuse thickening in which painful fissures may develop. This condition is called keratodermia plantaris and has variable causes. It may be a form of psoriasis, may be familial, or may be a nonspecific condition noted during various climatic changes. Treatment consists of softening the heel by warm foot soaks followed by massage with a lanolin salve. If the cornified layer is thick, it should be removed with a pumice stone or an emery board. Deep fissures may be treated by applying silver nitrate to them, which is momentarily painful but hastens healing. Antibiotics that are not prone to create a sensitive local absorption may be used when the fissures are infected.

ATHLETE'S FOOT

Athlete's foot is a fungus infection characterized by itchy, scaly lesions between the toes that frequently lead to fissure formation. Secondary infections are not uncommon. Prophylaxis by use of good foot hygiene is the preferred treatment, but once the foot is infected specific medications can be effectively applied.

SOFT TISSUE TUMORS

Tumors of soft tissues are rare and most often are tumors of tendon sheaths called ganglia. Being of tendon sheath origin they are rarely malignant and require excision only when they interfere with function or comfort. Nodules may appear in the plantar fascia in the arch of the foot that are the equivalent of Dupuytren's contracture in the palm. These are removed when they impair normal gait and should be biopsied to differentiate them from fibrosarcoma.

DIABETIC DERMATOLOGICAL COMPLICATIONS

When dealing with dermatological conditions of the foot the possibility of underlying diabetes must always be considered. The tissues of diabetics heal poorly and the vascular impairment often associated with diabetes causes ischemia and neuropathy. Proper foot hygiene in diabetes is imperative. With increasing longevity there is an increasing incidence of diabetes and vascular insufficiency and thus an increasing occurrence of diabetic neuropathy, ulcer, and gangrene. The foot is the major site of these manifestations.

No foot problem in the diabetic patient can be taken lightly. Paring a callus is a major procedure and the ingrown toenail is a serious lesion. The usually innocuous dermatitis is a burden in the diabetic.

The status of circulation must be established. Large vessel obstruction or impairment causes an absence of pulsations, coldness of the distal extremity, absence of hair over the dorsum of the toes, a subjective history of claudication, blanching of the elevated foot, and rubor of the dependent foot. Sympathectomy and endarterectomy offer some help in large vessel disease, but the care of the foot cannot await improvement of circulation. Proper care must precede and follow definitive treatment of the vascular occlusive disease.

Small blood vessel obstruction in diabetes is frequently accompanied by neuropathy which is considered to be related to changes in the vasa nervorum. The neuropathy decreases the skin sensation, impairs motor function to varying degrees and causes anhidrosis. The impaired sensation allows trauma to go unnoticed and ulcerations to exist without pain. Secondary infection and distal gangrene result frequently. Because half of the diabetic patients develop ulcers and gangrene which eventually require amputation, it is imperative that preventive measures be instituted early and energetically.

Trauma to the feet must be avoided. This means proper foot wear. Socks should not be too tight nor should they wrinkle. They should be washed until they can shrink no more and at this size should fit perfectly. The feet should be washed daily with soap and water then dried meticulously by "blotting" rather than rubbing. The spaces between the toes must be carefully dried then massaged with a lanolin cream to soften the skin. The toenails should be cut straight across to prevent ingrowing of the edges. If this is a difficult chore for the patient, it should be done by a podiatrist or a trained relative. The older patients should have periods of rest during the day with their shoes removed.

Improvement of circulation is best attained with exercise. This consists of putting the ankle and knee through their ranges of motion and the foot through inversion and eversion, and flexing the toes. These exercises should be done repeatedly during the day both when the patient is wearing shoes or is barefooted. The diabetic may restrict his walking because of claudication, but the patient should walk daily to the point of pain and *slightly further* for exercise. *Heat should never be applied di-*

rectly to the feet in an attempt to improve circulation. Reflex heating by applying heating pads to the lower abdomen or upper thighs is the only safe application of heat. Wool socks may be worn to bed but electric pads and hot-water bottles should be avoided.

Edema developing from any reason must be energetically treated by bed rest and exercise while in bed. The foot of the bed may be elevated slightly in the presence of edema, but elevating the legs too high or for long periods of time should be avoided in the presence of arterial insufficiency regardless of the extent of edema. Pressure bandages must be used with caution to ensure pressure that is even enough to compress the veins but will not cause arterial constriction. After the edema has decreased a well-fitted elastic hose is helpful as it applies pressure more evenly than the wrapped elastic bandage. Only if he is thoroughly educated and follows a closely supervised and regimented program does a diabetic have a chance to walk on two good feet in his later years.

BIBLIOGRAPHY

DeTakats, G.: Diabetic vascular disease. South. Med. J. 57:1143, 1964.

Giannestras, N. J.: Plantar Keratosis, Treatment by Metatarsal Shortening. J. Bone Jt. Surg. 48-A:727, 1966.

Lewin, P.: The Foot and Ankle, ed. 4. Lea & Febiger, Philadelphia, 1959.

Montgomery, R. M.: Dermatological Care of the Painful Foot. J. Bone Jt. Surg. 46-A:1129, 1964.

Whitehouse, F. W., and Block, M. A.: The Problem of the Diabetic Foot. J. Amer. Geriat. Soc. 12: 1045, 1964.

Index